Praise for *The Goddess Revolution*

'*In The Goddess Revolution, Mel inspires
reclaim our love of food... quitting diets 1
your body is the practice of lasting freedor*
Tara Stiles, bestselling author and founder of Strala

'*Mel Wells goes beyond the number on the scale, dress size or waistline.
She shows you how to get out of that body prison and step firmly and
forever into body, mind and spirit freedom.*'
Julie Montagu, health coach, bestselling author, yoga instructor and star of *Ladies of London*

'*Mel Wells is a light in the world. She has a great aura and an exuberant
personality. In her book The Goddess Revolution, Mel helps us break free
of judgement and guilt – especially around food and our body image. You
will find the tools in Mel's book to bring your life into balance, experience
vibrant energy and to Have The Best Day Ever!*'
David 'Avocado' Wolfe, author, lecturer, nutritionist, publisher, philanthropist, adventurer

'*Just like Mel herself, her writing is pure, powerful, real and beautiful.
This book will sway you into the hidden corner of your subconscious and
reveal who you really are. A must read for anyone who doesn't know she's
a Goddess... yet.*'
Tanya Maher, founder of Tanya's Cafe and author of *The Uncook Book*

'*If you're done with vicious eating cycles and want to get rid of the food
demons in your life, this book is for you! Mel is absolutely right, we are
all goddesses in our own unique way and it's time we embrace it... The
Goddess Revolution is empowering and inspiring, making it easy to heal
your relationship with food.*'
Liana Werner-Gray, bestselling author of *The Earth Diet*

'*Mel has such an inspirational message to help women fall back in love with
themselves! She writes with such integrity and love...*'
Madeleine Shaw, health coach and bestselling author of *Get the Glow*

'*I LOVED the book! I adored it... kept re-reading it all trip!*'
Angelica Malin, Editor-in-Chief, *About Time* magazine

'*The Goddess Revolution is a modern woman's guide to debunking the
social belief system we all grew up with. Thank you for creating this rebel
lady bible and sharing it with us!*'
Emily Nolan, Chief Empowerment Officer of emilynolan.com

'Mel Wells is like a big sister or BFF sharing her energy, passion and enthusiasm to make the tricky and hard-to-navigate terrain of a woman's relationship with food one of total pleasure...'
LISA LISTER, AUTHOR OF CODE RED AND LOVE YOUR LADY LANDSCAPE

"From the very first page you can feel love, in abundance, for the reader... The Goddess Revolution focuses on all areas of health, but almost prioritizes emotional and mental health which is what sets it apart from other health books.'
NATHALIE EMMANUEL, ACTRESS, HOLLYOAKS, GAME OF THRONES AND FAST & FURIOUS 7

'I simply ADORE Mel's approach. This is a woman who actually GETS what it's like to have an up-and-down relationship with your body, who has struggled with and OVERCOME emotional eating and self-sabotage, and who is also incredibly open about her experience.'
KAT LOTERZO, AUTHOR, SPEAKER AND SUCCESS MENTOR FOR KICKASS WOMEN ENTREPRENEURS

'Mel teaches you how to fall back in love with your body, ditch the diets for good and truly nourish your body from the inside out, so you can actually do what you were born to do... LIVE! Mel, thank you for inspiring me so much!'
STEPHANIE WARING, ACTRESS, HOLLYOAKS

'Mel is so incredibly inspiring... I really believe this book will help so many women... such a special book, written so beautifully, that could really change your life!'
HELEN FLANAGAN, CORONATION STREET ACTRESS AND REALITY STAR

'Mel bravely shares with us her personal battles and journey towards finding self-happiness. I can't recommend this book enough, especially if, like me, you were one of those people who let diets and the way you look control your day-to-day life.'
ASHLEY JAMES, PRESENTER, MODEL AND STAR OF MADE IN CHELSEA

'The Goddess Revolution makes you feel you're not alone with your thoughts about weight, body image or acceptance! It's about learning to love who you are and not to under- or overeat. We've all had the not eating and then the bingeing that follows... it's learning to find that balance and this book shows you that it's not impossible to do.'
LAUREN GOODGER, MODEL AND STAR OF THE ONLY WAY IS ESSEX

'I've known Mel for nearly 10 years. What I find most beautiful about her work is her desire to help others lead a happy, healthy life. She is so full of positive energy that anyone lucky enough to meet her or be around her is touched by her light! I'm so excited to read a book that I know has been a labour of love and will change so many women's lives...'
ISKRA LAWRENCE, INTERNATIONAL MODEL AND EDITOR OF RUNWAYRIOT.COM

the Goddess Revolution

The Goddess Revolution

Make Peace with Food, Love Your Body and Reclaim Your Life

Mel Wells

HAY HOUSE, INC.
Carlsbad, California • New York City
London • Sydney • Johannesburg
Vancouver • New Delhi

First published and distributed in the United Kingdom by:
Hay House UK Ltd, Astley House, 33 Notting Hill Gate, London W11 3JQ
Tel: +44 (0)20 3675 2450; Fax: +44 (0)20 3675 2451; www.hayhouse.co.uk

Published and distributed in the United States of America by:
Hay House Inc., PO Box 5100, Carlsbad, CA 92018-5100
Tel: (1) 760 431 7695 or (800) 654 5126
Fax: (1) 760 431 6948 or (800) 650 5115; www.hayhouse.com

Published and distributed in Australia by:
Hay House Australia Ltd, 18/36 Ralph St, Alexandria NSW 2015
Tel: (61) 2 9669 4299; Fax: (61) 2 9669 4144; www.hayhouse.com.au

Published and distributed in the Republic of South Africa by:
Hay House SA (Pty) Ltd, PO Box 990, Witkoppen 2068
info@hayhouse.co.za; www.hayhouse.co.za

Published and distributed in India by:
Hay House Publishers India, Muskaan Complex, Plot No.3, B-2,
Vasant Kunj, New Delhi 110 070
Tel: (91) 11 4176 1620; Fax: (91) 11 4176 1630; www.hayhouse.co.in

Distributed in Canada by:
Raincoast Books, 2440 Viking Way, Richmond, B.C. V6V 1N2
Tel: (1) 604 448 7100; Fax: (1) 604 270 7161; www.raincoast.com

A catalogue record for this book is available from the British Library.

ISBN: 978-1-78180-712-5

Interior images: Okea/Thinkstockphotos

Dedicated to my beautiful mum, Jackie,
a Goddess through and through.

Contents

Contents

god·dess

(gŏdĭs)

noun

1. A female being of supernatural powers or attributes, believed in and worshipped by a people.

2. A female being believed to be the source of life.

3. A woman who is in the process of learning to know, accept and love herself on all levels: mind, body and spirit. A woman who understands that she has unlimited capacity to make her life anything she wants. A woman who is inspired to give to those around her because of her sense of gratitude and abundance.

'Your body is precious.
It is our vehicle
for awakening.'

BUDDHA

From One Goddess to Another

Our stories around food, weight and body image are all so very personal. We keep them tight to our chests, for fear of being judged or misunderstood. Yet so many of us are secretly letting them rule our days, which in time allows them to rule our lives. Talking about how we feel around food, and living in our flawed bodies, can feel like we are baring our naked souls.

I'm sure, like me, you've seen those 'before and after' diet photos on social media. Transformation stories that compare the difference in body shape or size, and congratulate the dieter on her 'huge achievement, hard work and willpower'.

But... what if, despite losing weight, nothing really changed inside that woman's head, when it came to how she *felt* about herself?

What if she was still at war with her body, despite it changing physically due to a gruelling regime? What if she was still not at peace with what she saw in the mirror, despite celebrating such a 'win' with weight loss, and being commended by her trainer and fellow dieters? What if she still agonized every day over her food choices and criticized herself in every photo? Where would that leave her? Is that still a success story?

The real transformations that last for *life* are the game-changing, show-stopping, quantum shifts in mind-set – which in turn are reflected back at you in every area of your life. Not just your body shape or fat percentage.

No one woman's experience is the same as another around food or her body.

Whether a girlfriend recommended this book to you, you ordered it online or picked it up in a bookstore, I am so pleased that you did. You are on your own unique journey with food and your body, based on your experiences and conditioning, up to this very point of you picking up this book and deciding to start reading.

In this book, I'll share my personal revolution around food, weight and my body, and give you the life-changing tools and principles you need to break out of what may feel like body jail, for life.

I'll also be sharing a few of the stories from inspirational Goddesses who have joined the revolution and made quantum shifts too – way beyond what any diet club could compete with – real, raw transformational stories, where the change has happened from within. You might not relate so much to my story – but one of theirs might hit you so hard that you fall off your chair and get smacked awake.

Yep – this journey goes way deeper than celebrating a number on the scales or a size in the back of a dress.

You are not alone

Millions of women feel like they are living in a body that doesn't feel like theirs, while others are living day to day, consumed by dieting rules and obsessive thoughts around food and weight.

It's time we speak out and have those conversations around food, weight and body image that we have been keeping inside our own heads.

Through my own journey, my healing and my self-practice, I've discovered the key to finding total freedom around food and in my body.

It is now my life's work, to pass this on to you, and for you to be rewarded with waking up every day feeling absolutely comfortable in your own skin, free from rules, free from fear or guilt surrounding food and ready to create whatever you want from life – without being held back by how you feel about your body and your unwanted food patterns.

The Revolution is here, Goddess.

Part I

My Story

From Hating Myself Thin... to Loving Myself Healthy

'The wound is the place where the light enters you.'

Rumi

I am so passionate about healing women's relationship with food because it took me so long to heal my own.

My greatest fear was giving up my abusive and addictive relationship with food. It was my safety net, my best friend. It also nearly destroyed me. In a short space of time I went from a happy-go-lucky teen to a liar and a secret-keeper. I shied away from social situations, snapped at loved ones, felt disgusted at myself, hideously ashamed and embarrassed. But I was also in denial that I had any sort of problem.

I used food to numb my feelings, to punish myself, to reward myself. I used it to cover up so much of what was going on in my life that I didn't want to face or deal with. It was my comfort blanket, the thing I always turned to. I felt lost without it. I was so addicted to my destructive eating patterns that at times I felt like a drug user, in serious need of rehab.

Talking about it now is like describing a totally different person – a whole other life to the one I'm living now. Now I embrace myself in every way. I love and respect my body every day and wouldn't dream of abusing it. But even after years in recovery, I still feel as though I have a lifetime of making up to do.

Growing up, I felt like I had it all. I loved my life. I loved my friends. And it was fair to say I loved myself too.

Dieting never crossed my mind, the word wasn't even part of my vocabulary. My mum never dieted and I ate whatever I wanted – junk food mostly – and took part in sport and dance competitions every month, which I *loved*, and which kept me super-slim and *seemingly* healthy. (*Slim equals healthy, right?*)

At 16, things changed.

I went to a Performing Arts College to study acting, (*of course I did!*). From the outset the competition was palpable, and bitchy remarks and self-scrutiny were the norm. I was used to being a high achiever, but surrounded by other adolescent girls developing curves and critiquing their bodies, it wasn't long before I started to dim my light and ask, '*Who am I to be the one who is confident in my own skin? Who am I to dare to love myself?*'

I desperately wanted to make friends and to fit in, so when the other girls complained about being fat, I joined in too – pinching my belly and hips and pulling a face. When they started diets, I started one too.

But I couldn't do it by halves. Doing a well-known cereal diet with a friend turned into a competition of who could lose the most weight quickest, which turned into scrapping the cereal and becoming addicted to calorie-free soda and flavoured water, which soon escalated into ordering diet pills from the Internet – cue hot sweats, and uncontrollable shakes at night-time. But none of it mattered, starving didn't matter, I was now addicted to seeing my body shrink.

Somehow I was still getting top grades for my coursework and landing great roles in shows. But on the inside, I was at total war with myself – and as I lost pounds, I also lost my mojo, my spark, my personality, myself.

Looking back it's easy to see that what I was really searching for was the happiness and self-acceptance I'd lost. But I was convinced it came with a number. If I reached that number or size, I would suddenly feel empowered and confident again. I would suddenly not care what other people thought of me. I would get my mojo back. I would be able to live the life I wanted. But no way could I go after those dreams 'til I had achieved that perfect number first.

And so the war with myself continued...

What happened next took me completely by surprise: I landed a role in a major UK soap, *Hollyoaks*, and within a couple of weeks had moved my entire life up to an apartment in Liverpool to begin work.

It sounds like a dream. I was in a well-paid job, on TV every night and starting to be recognized when I went out. But the flipside told a different story. I was far away from home and living alone for the first time, and couldn't bear to watch myself on TV or see my picture emblazoned across the tabloids. I was 18, overwhelmed, alone and out of my depth.

Now instead of controlling what I ate, I lost all control. I started bingeing like I'd never seen or eaten food before. I was like a woman possessed. I didn't even taste what I was eating – I inhaled it like it was oxygen. Then, of course, the guilt would hit. I'd throw the food away and make myself sick 'til there were tears streaming down my face.

Sometimes I'd even go back to the bin like a feral cat to retrieve the leftover foods and carry on my pattern. Then I would make a plan to 'start again tomorrow' and starve myself for a few days – while making expeditions to the gym where I'd pound the treadmill 'til I was so bored I could cry – to 'make up for it' or 'reverse' my binge.

I remember thinking, I'm living the dream
I always had growing up – I've got a
major part on a regular TV show – so
why do I feel so empty and unhappy?

Try as I might to distract myself with nights out and frenzied shopping splurges to fill the void, I felt an overwhelming sense of loneliness and emptiness. It was like there was something missing and my food addiction filled the gap.

I saw a couple of counsellors during that time – but chose not to let them in. A part of me still wanted to stay in the little hell I had created – it was comfortable and safe. The more I told myself I needed fixing, the more I gave myself permission to keep repeating the same patterns. I was telling myself the same thing over and over again: *This is who I am. I will have to live like this for the rest of my life and nobody can save me.*

When my character was written out of the show around the time of a new producer arriving, I was devastated. But in hindsight I believe it was a higher power looking out for me. I wasn't coping at all and had completely lost any sense of who I was.

When the Hollywood producers weren't banging down my door, I started modelling. I loved travelling every day to photo shoots – it was loads of fun – but, of course, it came with more body pressures.

I would show up to jobs and if my measurements weren't perfect, as they 'should' be, I was sent home and replaced. And when I did get the job, seeing airbrushed photos reinforced my belief that my body needed 'fixing' to look good enough.

More than anything I believed more
and more that my body needed to be
perfect or just shrink a little bit more.

What happened next completely shook my world and woke me up out of my self-obsessed existence.

During Christmas of 2011, my beloved Dad was diagnosed with stage four cancer and given four months to live. I can remember being in the room with him when we were told. That moment changed everything, and all three of us – my brother Charlie, Dad and I – squeezed each other's hands before crumbling and holding each other, shaking. *Four months* to spend with our amazing father before his time was up and he was taken from us for ever.

My dad was this jolly, big personality and exuberant character, who charmed the socks off everyone he met. He would walk into a room and everyone would love his energy! He had this amazing aura – I was so proud to call him my dad. And I was definitely his number-one girl.

In many ways he always took great care of himself, but when it came to his health it was bottom of his priorities. 'Life's too short to be healthy,' he would laugh when I suggested he maybe cut down on the bacon and sausages. I didn't know a great deal about nutrition back then, but I had read every diet book on the shelf and knew he wasn't doing himself any favours. He was overweight, liked rich food and wine, and did no exercise. (*Perhaps, if he could have exercised in his best suit he would have tried.*)

Those last four months with Dad were a complete blur. Every day I would break down in tears, and scream and pray for help. Ryan, my partner at the time, was my rock throughout it all – and

I am so grateful to him for being there for me. I did everything possible to spend as much time with Dad, making him feel more important, more loved and more cared for than anyone else in the world.

To my surprise, he began to seek out books on cancer. 'I want to know about this bastard thing that's killing me,' he said, which made me remember a book someone had once recommended: *The China Study*, the most comprehensive nutrition and health study ever conducted. I devoured the book and it blew my mind that with every form of cancer or disease – the answer to prevention was simple: less processed food, fewer animal products and more plants, a more alkaline way of life.

I started encouraging Dad to eat more of the right foods. But sadly, by this time, he was unable to eat much at all and was on shakes and meal replacements. I felt like I had uncovered the world's best-kept secret – but all too late to save him. In April 2012, he passed away peacefully and became my angel.

The grief of losing him made it even harder to control my eating, but finding a resolution became more urgent and more purposeful. I had never felt more called to share a message with the world and decided to start training in nutrition to become a health coach. I didn't see it as a new career – all I knew was I was hungry for more information, and to help spread this message far and wide about cancer prevention, and in turn hope to heal myself too.

The Missing
Vitamin L(ove)

I began spreading the message far and wide about the health benefits of plant-based living and started creating vegan recipes to help the world combat disease. It was wonderful!

But did this actually heal my relationship with food and end the war I had on my body?

No... actually it didn't.

I now had a better understanding of nutrition and healthy living, but I also had a brand new set of rules to abide by when it came to food – essentially, a new perfect diet to use and abuse.

Being vegan didn't stop me hating my body and messing around with calories. I was eating better foods, but still with the same bad habits. Instead of bingeing on refined sugar, I was bingeing on medjool dates and nuts.

I began to think that no amount of new nutrition information could heal my relationship with food. I was searching for a miracle that would make everything fall into place and make me feel happy about being in my body. It took a while to realize that I was looking in all the wrong places.

Being a mum has always been one of the single most important things to me. I have always known that I wanted to have children, but when my partner and I started to have serious discussions about having a baby, it suddenly hit me like a ton of bricks: *How on earth was I going to be a good role model to my kids? How could I possibly carry on this way of eating and talking down to my body, and pass on this warped mind-set to an innocent child?*

I wasn't even sure whether I'd be able to conceive, given how much I had messed around with my insides. Not only that but I was so obsessed with how my body looked. How on earth would I deal with being pregnant and losing the baby weight quickly? It was bound to send me insane. Would I have been trying to do a juice cleanse or strict fast the day after popping a baby out? Probably. And even I could see how messed up that would be.

I decided that something needed to change *drastically*, if I wanted the responsibility of starting a family and being a healthy role model to my kids. I made a promise to myself to quit my behaviour, and make friends with my body: to make her a healthy environment to grow a baby. I decided to have one full year of being 'healthy' not 'skinny' – then I would be ready to conceive.

I started focusing on *healing* my body, exercising for strength and fitness and *fun* rather than to burn calories. I stopped scrutinizing myself in the mirror every day and stopped trying to follow strict rules around food.

I threw the rulebook away and began to connect and listen to my body again.

At first, it was shaky. I didn't trust myself and was terrified of gaining weight. But I was determined to heal my body, so I threw away the scales, which I had been so reliant on for validation every morning. What happened in time was *miraculous*. It felt like I was coming home to my body after so many years of fighting her.

I became more present with my friends and family. I stopped being so on edge in social situations involving food. I started to cook more than just diet meals – and actually find *joy* from food again – something I hadn't let be an enjoyment or pleasure in my life since I was at school.

I had taken on being skinny as a *full-time job*, and it was such a relief to surrender it and resign!

I began to develop my message promoting an anti-dieting approach to health. And the more women I spoke to, the more I realized how many of us are fighting a seemingly never-ending battle with food and our body. It is an epidemic.

> *I thought I was fighting a secret war that nobody else would understand – I had no idea how many other women in the world were fighting similar battles.*

Since I made this shift, I've developed many lessons and tools to help women everywhere fall back in love with their lives. More in love with themselves, and more at peace with food and their bodies than they ever thought possible! And yes – through this process – astonishingly, I've lost any excess weight I was carrying from my old bad binge habits. I realized it didn't have to be such a struggle. But way better, I regained my *life* back, and actually became *happy* again in my body *regardless* of what I weighed.

The tools and principles I now teach are those I've learned through my own struggles, and those of my clients, and that's exactly what I am here to share with you in this book. In the following pages you'll discover new mind-set hacks to help you break destructive food patterns and appreciate your body, so that you too can be the healthiest and happiest you've ever been.

The revolution is here, and I'm so excited for you to join me.

No amount of dieting or new nutrition information can make you love your body. That is the work of the Goddess.

Part II

The Perfect Diet

A culture fixated on female thinness is not an obsession about female beauty, but an obsession about female obedience. Dieting is the most potent political sedative in women's history; a quietly mad population is a tractable one.

NAOMI WOLFE

Diet: A Way of Life?

I asked a diverse group of women what thoughts and feelings came up for them when I said the word **'diet'**. Here's a snippet of what they said to me:

* rules
* weighing
* self-loathing
* skinny
* inadequacy
* restriction
* meal plans
* deprivation
* calories
* willpower
* abs
* hunger
* scales
* guilt
* salad
* failure
* counting
* bingeing
* starting again on Monday

'Diet', originally derived from the Greek *dialita*, means 'a way of life'.

Call me crazy, but none of the above sound like an appealing way of life from where I'm sat.

The New Holy Grail

Millions of women around the world are searching for the perfect diet, but what is it that we're really seeking?

We want a diet that will fulfil us, support us, energize us, make us happy, make our skin glow and make the pounds drop off effortlessly.

Why is this perfect diet so damn hard to come across? And more to the point, why are we all so *utterly useless* at sticking to diets anyway? Wouldn't life *be so much better if* we could just get our food sorted out and find the perfect set of rules to follow so we can focus on the more important stuff?

Our quest for the perfect diet is intertwined with our quest for the perfect physique, which has us looking to punish our body for not being good enough, so we start thinking…

Maybe my food combining is all off? Maybe I'm eating too much healthy fat? Maybe I should cut out all sugar for three weeks? Maybe I'm eating too much fruit, or eating too late at night?

Diet culture has sucked so much joy out of eating that we now use food in ways that it was never intended. We've forgotten that food is essentially there to sustain us, to nourish us, to be enjoyed and loved. We've neglected our *relationship* with food so much that we just grab things and shove them into our mouths without a second thought. We don't even experience food's tastes and textures before it's swallowed and we're on to the next thing.

Have you ever got up really early in the morning, crawled into the car like a zombie and then suddenly you're at work, with no real recollection of how you got there?

We do this with food *all the time*.

Now think about your body and how you treat it.

How you REALLY treat it.

With your thoughts, with your words, with your feelings and actions.

We have got so used to being disconnected from our body – it is just being lugged around with us all day like a backpack. We chuck things in without really thinking. We eat foods without even really understanding what they are, or where they come from, or what ingredients they contain.

Throughout this book you'll often hear me refer to your body as 'she' or 'her' rather than 'it'. Your body represents the Goddess and I want you to start thinking of your body as a separate, female entity that deserves your worship and respect.

Ask yourself.

* Do you respect her?

* Do you look at her with disgust?

* Do you berate her?

* Do you tell her with your thoughts she isn't good enough?

* Do you slow down and listen to her?

* Do you trust her?

* Do you try to manipulate her with rules?

* Are you loving towards her?

* Are you grateful for your body, or have you totally abandoned and disconnected from her entirely?

Your relationship with food and your relationship with your body are intertwined. But are you connected to either? Or have you abandoned both?

> **Contrary to what the diet industry would have you think, food is not there for you to be at war with. It is not supposed to be the enemy.**

You need food to nourish your body, to empower you, and to allow you to take care of yourself and your beautiful body, of which you only have one. The more you diet, the less connected you will feel to your body and your food. The further away from yourself you will be.

Your Relationship with Food

You can eat all the kale, quinoa and raw hemp protein in the world, but if you're still obsessing over that slice of pizza you ate last weekend, that's not healthy. Don't sacrifice a healthy mind-set in the pursuit of a healthy body.

Good nutrition is so important. Making sure you're eating fresh vegetables, fruits, leafy greens, good fats and good-quality proteins is vital to having a healthy body. BUT, it's not the whole conversation, Goddess.

Yes – I'm afraid to say that all these conversations about nutrition and diets are missing a vital component of what it takes to be healthy and live in a body you love. The missing link is:

Understanding your relationship with food.
The soul of who you are as an eater.

This is absolutely vital for lasting change, and the main reason that short-term diet changes do not and will not ever work for us.

Nutritionists tell us, 'Eat this. Don't eat that.' These evaluations are based on nutritional values, calories, grams, vitamins and nutrient content, and these are the rules you should follow. And all of these articles, books and experts are correct in their studies, I'm sure. There's no denying that if they have spent 20 years studying nutrition, they should probably know a lot about what they're talking about.

But it's just not the **whole** conversation.

Nutrition is not discussing your thoughts, feelings, emotions around before and after you eat. Nutrition is not discussing the other moving components of your life, your relationships, your work life and how *that* affects your eating. Nutrition just scratches the surface of the whole story you've got going on here.

> *Food itself is usually not the problem*
> *at all – it's just the symptom.*

How you use food can point to an area of your life that needs urgent attention. That may be a relationship, your home environment, your career, your finances, your spirituality, or how you're expressing or suppressing yourself every day.

Nutrition doesn't embrace the psychology behind your food-making decisions, or what you feel in your heart and soul before you decide what to eat.

So if you're basing all your food choices on nutritional science only – chances are, you're not seeing the bigger picture.

You could be eating a big bowl of salad, but if you're stuffing it into your mouth frantically, so that you don't have to deal with the upset in your relationship, does that still make it healthy?

Kale can be a weapon too, y'know.

Sure, it's not as much of a weapon of mass destruction as a cheeseburger or hotdog – but any food can be damaging to you if you eat it with a certain approach.

**It's not all about the food any more.
It never really was. It's about your
entire mind-set around eating.**

When I was a serial binge eater, I was still doing what I thought
was my **best** to eat healthily. This saw me bingeing on entire trays
of medjool dates, raw vegan chocolate, huge selection bags of
dried fruit and nuts, and getting through entire tubs of almond or
peanut butter in a week.

All healthy foods! All part of my healthy diet! But I was still
bingeing like crazy on them and losing complete control.

It was totally emotional eating and I was mindlessly shovelling
it into my body, completely disconnected from how she was
feeling or what I didn't want to deal with in that moment. (Moving
locations, being in an unfulfilling career, longing for more intimacy
and affection, desperate to feel understood.)

To an outsider, I had a healthy diet, sure. But my *relationship*
with food was far from healthy.

**You came into this world with a purpose,
and your relationship with food is here to
guide you on how to fill in the blanks.**

Instead of being angry with your body, or angry at your relationship
with food, stop trying to beat it into submission – surrender the fight.
Treating your relationship to food with attacking, negative thoughts
will never lead to a beautiful ending.

Relationships need to be nurtured in order to grow and
blossom into something beautiful. Accept exactly where you are,
and trust that it is exactly where you are meant to be. Open your
mind to listening to your body and being honest with how you
treat her.

We live in a world that disconnects us from our body's wisdom, and gives us so many external distractions and reasons to avoid looking within ourselves. When you shut out the chaos and really pay attention to YOU, your life and your body – as a Goddess and as an eater – what you discover may surprise you.

You may have huge light-bulb moments go off. You may have events from your past rear their head that you didn't expect you would ever have to deal with again. Don't shut these down. Instead, welcome them to the discussion with an open mind, and do your best to listen to what they may be trying to tell you.

Pay attention

In order truly to dive deep into our relationship with food, we must become masters at observing ourselves. Your relationship with food is here to teach you and, if you are a willing student, you can learn so many life-changing, invaluable lessons. So observe yourself like the top student at school. You are at the school of YOU.

You are here to fall in love with yourself.
You are here to win the battle within your head.
You are here to accept yourself fully
and let the love flood in.

But first you have to learn to observe yourself – with patience and kindness.

Watch your habits closely and carefully observe your behavioural patterns before and after eating. Observe how you feel in every moment. Ask yourself: How do I feel before eating? What are the reasons behind my eating?

Really get honest about why you chose to eat. Did you really want to or were you pressured into eating by someone else? Or was it a habit you were going along with mindlessly? Was an emotion driving you to eat or was it your body's natural appetite? If you don't know – get to know.

Your Relationship with Food Is Your Teacher – Be a Willing Student

Respect your teacher just as you would at school. If you don't pay attention to the lessons your relationship with food is trying to teach you, they will keep showing up, year after year after year – until you sit up and actually listen. What you resist will persist.

Every unwanted pattern, or eating challenge, has a lesson within it. Each bad food habit that you perceive to be a problem carries a wisdom and hidden message – and it is your job to discover exactly what that is.

When you start observing your thoughts, rather than passively going along with the same patterns, you'll start to see how you have the power to change those thoughts, and therefore your mind-set around food, and everything else in your life entirely.

A fish can't see water because it's in it.
Sometimes you can't see your thoughts and
habits because you're just so engulfed in them.

Start by observing your thought processes and feelings like an outsider looking in. Study your feelings and observe your thoughts. It's important not to judge your thoughts – just breathe and observe. Be curious. Be inquisitive.

When you start doing this, you'll be tuning in to your body in a brand new way and connecting your thought processes to your actions around food. Ask yourself

- What can I do to best support myself right now?

- What is my favourite excuse to use, or way in which I sabotage myself?

- What patterns am I noticing?

Don't judge what comes back. Just observe it, and say to yourself, 'How very curious that is – I must investigate more!'

Your Relationship with Food Is Unique to YOU

There are no short-cuts here – but you know that, because you know diets haven't really worked for you in the long run.

If you have a challenging relationship with food – trust innately that you are absolutely here to start healing it, to connect the dots and to nurture it back to where it belongs. Your relationship with food is here to help you uncover the hidden messages behind your habits – and why?

You are here to live a fulfilled and soulful life!

Your unwanted eating habits may be screaming at you that a particular area of your life is not at peace. If you listen to and observe what they are trying to teach you, they will be able to guide you in the direction of the most soulful, beautiful life you could possibly imagine.

Could that *be* any more exciting?

This is why I have so many clients end our work together, and weeks later, send me an email saying:

> *'Mel! You won't believe it! I have finally ended my awful and unfulfilling relationship with that guy, and I feel so much more connected to myself and happy!'*

Or

> *'Since we ended our work, I've realized how miserable*
> *my job makes me, so I've decided to finally bite the*
> *bullet and quit my job to follow my dreams instead!'*

It's not about the food any more at all. It's about self-worth. Food, as I said before, is just the symptom.

When you uncover the messages behind what's driving your emotional eating, weight gain or unwanted food habits, the possibilities are endless. You lose the weight you didn't want – and you become free to live the life of your dreams – a life of purpose, soul fulfilment and magic. Not only that – but you are doing it with a body that you love living in!

How to Know If You're a Yo-yo Dieter

Just in case you're suffering with a little denial, as I used to, let me give you a hand. Classic traits of yo-yo dieters include:

- 'Starting again' on Monday.

- Tracking everything you eat.

- Always being lured in by the next hot diet.

- Always buying the next new diet book.

- Always wanting to know what people eat.

- Always wanting to know what people weigh.

- Always wanting to know what diet people are on.

- Always telling people you're 'off track right now' or 'need to get back on track'.

- Always deciding to cut out something new.

- Always comparing your body to other women's bodies.

- Always knowing exactly what you weigh.

* Defining your weeks into 'good' and 'bad' days.

* Striving to 'eat clean' in the week only to binge over the entire weekend.

I know all this because I yo-yo dieted like a pro and for a few years, I would lose and gain the same 30lbs over and over *and over again* using various different methods.

Every Monday I had a new rule, or a new meal plan (meal plans are just diets in disguise). By Tuesday I felt like a saint. Like, *so* virtuous right now. By the middle of the week I was bored and planning my weekend binge. By Friday I was scoffing like I'd never seen food before in my life, and by Sunday I had eaten myself to the point of self-loathing and often into physical pain.

Sunday night I would then form my new plan. A new set of rules. This week, *this week it would be different.* I would be *even* stricter. Or cut out even more food groups. Monday morning I would wake up, weigh myself – hate myself – and start over.

I fooled myself that if I could *just find the right set of rules*, or *just have enough discipline* to make it through a few weeks to start seeing results, I would have the body of my dreams, and therefore the life of my dreams. After all, I couldn't possibly achieve anything I wanted while my body wasn't where I wanted it to be, right?

My life couldn't truly begin, until I had fixed my body first.

When Food Talks to You...

Sounds crazy – right? But you feel like food is *actually talking to you*. From inside the cupboards. From inside the fridge. You feel like it is calling your name. Making you go and eat it. You're fooled into thinking *you're* the one controlling your food – but if you're honest you know it's the other way round. Your every thought is spent thinking about food, your next meal, your rules.

And the food is speaking to you, urging you to break all these carefully laid-out rules. You feel out of control around food. You feel like food literally runs your life – runs your mind.

But starting a new diet will never change that.

Why?

It is a *direct* result of the diet industry itself.

I often felt like I was so addicted to food, I used to wonder if this was how drug addicts felt. After all, it's the same thing right? Using food, alcohol, drugs, sex or whatever your chosen vice, to numb yourself and 'cope' with areas of your life that don't feel balanced.

The difference is that alcohol and substance abusers can go to rehab. They can practise abstinence and 'get sober'. They can, if they put their mind to it, go cold turkey and 'quit'. We can't do this with food. When we try to practise abstinence from our food addictions, it is a diet. This, of course, worsens our relationship with food. Which makes the addiction an even greater force. Oh dear.

After all – it's not like we can abstain from food forever. We gotta eat.

We therefore have no other choice but to find a way to live with food in harmony. Food is not going anywhere, any time soon! Attention to your relationship with food is key and ditching the diet mind-set is crucial, if you want to completely lose those unwanted crazy eating patterns and finally understand how it feels to be 'normal' with your food and live in a healthy, happy body for life, without shame or judgement.

You only ever feel 'out of control' around food
because you have been desperately trying
TO control your food in the first place.

Is Food Your Frenemy?

Food gets it.

She takes you in her arms and hugs you, at the end of a stressful day. Or when your love life takes a tumble… You have good times with food. Food makes you feel so happy.

Your friendship is a hit of pleasure and comfort at the same time. She makes you feel grounded and safe. She is your entertainment when you're bored. When you need to fill time, food is there.

When you need to be distracted, you know for sure you can rely on food to do that. Or when you need to be calmed down – food will do that. She's got your back.

But… you know that one day – at the flip of a switch – this 'friend' is out to get you.

Without warning, food sends you into a downward spiral of **self-loathing**. She makes you feel **unworthy, un-beautiful, unlovable**. She makes you feel small.

Food takes great pleasure in knocking you down a peg or two. She tells you that you're **not enough** as you are, that you should change your body before you're allowed to be happy.

You hate the discomfort – the pain, the guilt and shame. But for some reason, she convinces you that you deserve it. And there you are again – at war with yourself once more. It seems food wasn't your friend after all.

Toxic relationships and friendships do NOT serve you.

Either you walk away from the relationship
or you heal it with trust, respect and love.

You cannot heal a toxic relationship by putting more hate and fight into it. It just doesn't work. And, since you can't walk away from your relationship with food, it looks like you're here to start healing it.

This love–hate, Jekyll-and-Hyde thing you have going on with food… **is slowly destroying your spirit.** *Nothing loving can be created when we allow food to trigger our self-loathing.*

The way to make friends again with food *is to make friends with yourself and your body first.*

You have the power to make your friendship with food a loving one.

A joyful, balanced, two-sided one, where you win. You can love food and love yourself both at the same time.

But if you want to do this, you have to stop the fight.

You only truly win when you stop fighting.

And instead, start loving.

Goddess Emma
. . . .

'Now there's no guilt or shame around food. I listen to what my body wants and give it to her in abundance.'

I'd been overweight my whole life and, although it sometimes isolated me growing up, I knew that I could always eat my feelings and tried not to let it get to me too much. That is, until 2013 when, after having three beautiful girls, I knew it was time to do something about my weight because I wanted to be healthy for them.

I'd tried diets before but this time I joined a slimming club and a gym and stuck with it. I lost 3st in the first year, but then it started to get harder and it no longer felt healthy so I left. I spent the next year yo-yoing between different plans, other diet clubs/counting calories/macro counting/low-carb/Paleo – searching for the one perfect thing that would help me keep losing weight.

On the outside I pretended to be fine but inside I was crumbling. I was trying to control the one thing that shouldn't ever be controlled and it was taking a toll on the rest of my life. I know I was pretty difficult to live with during this time. I was addicted to weighing myself several times a day, wouldn't eat out unless I had planned it meticulously, and felt guilty if I went off plan and then spent days trying to undo the damage. I was a hamster on a wheel that couldn't get off. I felt stuck, fed up, sad. I knew I wasn't showing my beautiful girls the right way to live life but I didn't know how to stop. Until that is, I found Mel.

Now I love my body and am proud of her for the strength she has and what she can do. I adore the fact she's given us three beautiful girls. OK, I'm still a little overweight but it's not a big deal because now I'm healthy, and the gym and lifting weights is changing my body immensely, and I love it!

Don't get me wrong – sometimes I choose to give her too much chocolate or wine, but the thing is now that's my choice and I own it – and there are no rules to follow apart from my own. I'm free and it's amazing.

Now I have the confidence to follow my dreams, and I'm going to grab every opportunity that comes my way.

Diet Culture: Thinks about body looking a certain way... eats three cupcakes, beans on toast, a whole tray of cookies, kitchen sink and a small village.

No Diet Is Going to Save You! You Are the One Here to Do That

Here's the deal, Goddess.

It's not *you* that keeps failing the diet, OK?

Diets don't work, period.

They are *designed* not to work and 95 per cent of women who go on diets and lose weight, gain all the weight back within a year.

Why? The diet is not fundamentally getting to the root cause of your unwanted eating habits or body hating. The diet is barely scratching the surface, and long term is actually doing more harm than good.

The few per cent that have the big weight-loss transformations and *do* keep it off for life are the ones learning to connect again with their bodies. The ones scrapping the rules – and instead creating healthy lifestyles they love.

It's not *you* that doesn't get it, or can't fix yourself. You are not alone. And you do not need to glorify 'willpower'.

Willpower

There is only so far you can go when you rely solely on your own strength, willpower and discipline to do the work.

'If only I had better willpower – I'd be so good at sticking to my diet. I'd have this diet thing *nailed!*'

'I'm on the Paleo diet – I just need better discipline.'

'If I just had better willpower I'd be flying!'

What if I told you it's not about willpower or discipline at all?

What if I told you, having *'not very good willpower'* could actually be one of the best things ever to happen to you?

Having 'no willpower', actually means you're connecting and listening to your body when it calls. It means that when your body wants to rebel against your rules you're able to hear her loud and clear, and you want to listen to her.

We are not supposed to be following rules and disconnecting emotionally from our body.

This is why meal plans don't last. It's just a set of rules to follow. Most of us are emotional, intuitive creatures and will eventually want to break these rules – whether we know it fully or it's a subconscious desire to sabotage ourselves.

How do you feel *after* you break these rules you have around food?

Awful? Like you failed? Like you're 'off track'? Like you need to make up for it or reverse it ASAP? Or, you say, 'Oh well, may as well write off the rest of the day (or the weekend) and start afresh on Monday.' (*Diets always start on Monday, right?*)

Here's what actually happened:

Your body's natural intuition kicked in and said, *'I don't like these rules. I don't want to follow them any more. I know better.'* And all you did was paid attention and listened. But you probably went overboard because you're so used to being disconnected and have glorified the feeling of being 'in control'.

There are many reasons we are called to eat, so it's highly unlikely a meal plan or set of rules will take into account:

* Your cravings

* Your social schedule

* Your hormones

* Your lifestyle

* Your relationships

* Your physical activity

* How tired you are

* Your mental state of wellbeing

* Your hydration

* Your body type

* Your genetics

* Your climate

This cycle of starting and failing diets can feel like it's never-ending – and that's because that's exactly what they are designed to do. Diets are designed for you to fail them so that you come back and give it another go.

Your body winds up being so confused with all the ups and downs. First you're trying so hard to have strong discipline and willpower, then the second your intuition kicks in and you break those rules you beat yourself up for it and end up in a spiral of self-hate. And this makes you feel worse than before and more at war with your body than you did to start with.

But *still...* you start again the following Monday telling yourself that *this time, this time you'll have more discipline and better willpower.*

Imagine how it would feel to be free from rules and completely connected to your body at all times. You would never binge, you would never overeat and you would never need to start a new diet again. Imagine simply being in a constant, calm conversation with your body and how she feels.

Our biggest fear about what will happen when we 'listen to our body' is 'that we will just end up eating junk food all day – get unhealthy and gain weight. Our biggest fear is that listening to our body will lead to us eating all the 'wrong' foods, and in turn feeling unhappy and fat.

**Diet culture leads us to believe that we
are useless without rules and structure.**

But you don't need rules and structure. You need to surrender and trust your body – but you also need a good education around nutrition, healthy living and how to take care of yourself and how to listen properly. You need to understand the difference between emotional cravings and real hunger cravings.

The truth is most people have no idea how amazing their body can actually feel, when they are nourishing her properly, listening and connecting – every day of the week.

When you develop the right mind-set around your food and body the two become so beautifully in tune that you really do *know* what it wants to be fed, in order to feel the best it can possibly feel.

You stop being drawn to the rubbish and start eating what will make your body feel most amazing. Sometimes you want green juice. Sometimes you want chocolate.

*Honour your body – she is much wiser
than you give her credit for.*

There is a divine connection between your mind, your food and your body – and once you master it, it will serve you for life. And you will laugh in the face of new diets that try and tempt you away.

You may think right now that your body is craving junk. You may have kidded yourself that you're 'addicted to sugar'. It's more likely, however, that you have become trapped in a pattern of unwanted habits that are being driven by your emotions – *not* sugar itself. Your healthiest, happiest body does not crave sugar. She craves an abundant lifestyle full of the vitamins and minerals she needs to function at her very best potential, to support you for life.

Good Days, Bad Days, the Track and the Wagon

Stop judging your days by putting them into categories of 'good' or 'bad'.

Stop labelling yourself as being either 'on track' or 'off track', or similarly 'on the wagon' or 'off the wagon'.

Scrap the track.
Scrap the wagon.

Life is a constant stream of choices. This includes choices around food. The track and the wagon are an illusion. You've created them as a way of judging yourself based on your choices and the pressure you have put on yourself to stay between certain lines.

When you take ownership over all of your choices, you won't feel the need to write an entire day off as a 'bad' day.

If you've made one food choice today that wasn't true to how you want to feel, and your body didn't love it? That's OK. It happens! You're human. Learn from it, and move on. And make your next choice a more positive, intuitive one.

> **Be in a constant state of learning from your own body and what she tells you. You are a student of yourself.**

When you screw up, skip a
workout or eat a meal not in
tune with how you want to feel
in your body, it doesn't make
you a bad person.
It makes you human.
Learn from it and move on.

Control vs. Intuition

As children, we're not taught to manipulate our food. We aren't taught to avoid carbs and watch out for fat content, and we certainly aren't taught to count calories.

But somewhere along the way, we've been led to believe that we need to have a plan in place with our food – to live by a certain label, diet or set of rules. This makes you feel like you're in control and you've got your shit together, right?

The opposite of control is surrender.
Trust your own intuition.
Your intuition is your greatest gift.
Don't ignore it.

The truth is most of us simply don't trust our body to make the right decisions. We think that if we don't manipulate our food in some way, then we'll just laze around all day eating sugary crap for the rest of our lives.

We *know* this isn't how to feel good. We *know* that's not what we want. But we live in fear of this, so we turn to looking for rules to regulate us.

❖ Why do we need the control?

❖ What are you struggling to control already?

❖ Where in your life do you feel out of control?

We only ever feel 'out of control' around food when we have tried desperately *to* control it. If you stopped trying to control it you would, in turn, never feel 'out of control'.

Embrace the messiness of life, and stand up to what you are struggling with. Ask yourself why food is being used as an attempt to control certain parts of your life. The answers do not lie in another diet or meal plan. The answers will be found when you get brutally honest with yourself and ask questions about YOU.

Food is not the problem – it's the symptom.

What would happen if we released the need to control?

Come Back to
Your Body

Your body is dying for you to come home.
Your body is desperate to reconnect.
Your body is waiting for you to come back to her.
Your body never abandoned you or left you.
Your body is yours for life. Yes – let that sink in.
You have this one vessel for the rest of your life.
Your home. You don't get to swap her.
So how have you been treating the home that you live in?
Have you been ignoring her?
Disrespecting her?
Fuelling her with self-hate, punishment and guilt?
Inhaling food without even tasting it or allowing it to digest?
Come home to your body.
Make friends and make her feel loved.
She never abandoned you.
She's waiting for you.

You Are Not Broken

You do not need fixing.
You are not different.
You are special, but you are not special.
We are all the same.
We are all whole.
We are all perfect, because of our beautiful imperfections.

......

When you've been a long-term dieter – or struggled with your relationship with food – you truly believe that *your body* is different from everyone else's. You believe that *you are broken* or something is intrinsically wrong with you. I know this because I believed it for years.

You may have toxic limiting beliefs that you are unlovable, unworthy, un-beautiful, because of the imperfections of your body, or how it looks when you stand naked in front of the mirror, prodding it. You may believe that everyone else gets to be happy now – but you can't. You don't deserve to. Not 'til you've fixed your body.

You probably have a bunch of stories about your body that you tell yourself. You convince yourself that you're special – you're broken – your body is different from everyone else's and you need to implement a ton of rules or spend your life searching for the perfect plan that will make you happy.

I'm sorry to be harsh – but this is all a complete crock of shit.

Don't worry. You're not a bad person. You're just used to the way diet culture has made you feel about yourself.

- Diets constantly reinforce the idea that you need fixing.

- Diets instil a belief in you that you need to fix your body before you're allowed to be happy.

We allow ourselves to be dominated by these thoughts, and we even surrender to the fact that we will never truly be OK. Food will always be a struggle. I'm here to tell you the opposite. Freedom and happiness can be *yours for life* – and you never need to diet again. The sooner you tear up the rulebook, the sooner you can be happy and truly start to reclaim your life.

The scales will only tell you the numerical value of your effect on gravity. They will not tell you how beautiful you are, how loved you are, or how amazing you are.

When I've Lost 10lbs I'll...

Life is short. Don't miss out on 95 per cent of your life just to weigh 5 per cent less.

Don't look back in 20 years wishing you'd taken more chances, allowed yourself to go on those crazy adventures, told someone how you feel, wore that amazing dress – asked that person out...

Those extra few pounds you may be carrying are not in your way. Don't let them stop you from living the life of your dreams.

Those extra few pounds may not fit into your made-up idea of what 'perfection' looks like, but they actually represent your *life*, and most likely where your body naturally wants to be. They represent your freedom, your ability to forgive and love yourself, your spontaneity and your fun.

Those unforgettable memories...

Meals out at gorgeous new restaurants... That cake your grandma is famous for baking and loves to surprise you with... The champagne you popped to celebrate your friend's new job... That romantic date night with your lover... The pizza you shared while adventuring in a new city... That bottomless brunch catching up with your favourite girlfriends...

One of the biggest issues with diet culture is that you end up telling yourself the same old story: *'If I just struggle now for a while, then I'll be allowed to be happy and enjoy those celebrations in life, later.'*

❖ *Then* I'll have the body so I can start living the life I want.

❖ *Then* I'll have the confidence to go on dates.

❖ *Then* I'll go after that job promotion.

❖ *Then* I'll have that photo shoot.

❖ *Then* I'll book that holiday and buy bikinis.

❖ *Then* I'll buy that cute outfit I want...

We deny ourselves pleasure and happiness until we have what we consider is the perfect body. The big issue with this, of course, is it means that literally millions of us around the world are *waiting* to lose weight before we allow ourselves to live our lives. Trapped in a never-ending cycle of diets that don't work.

Who do you know that lost a lot of weight on a diet and then lived happily ever after at complete peace with her body and food?

Most likely, if you know anyone who has had short-term success on a 'diet' and lost weight, she is still not at peace with her body. She may still berate herself in the mirror, she may still feel the need to stick to rules around food and put different foods into boxes – by way of points, sins or calories, and punish herself for going against the system that previously worked so well for her.

Most women don't simply do a diet, finish a diet and then live in happiness and freedom for the rest of their lives. More likely we either struggle to reach an end goal – then wonder why we're still unhappy when we get there – or start a diet, fail about 20 times, then give up altogether and sink into a black hole of self-loathing, telling ourselves, '*I just don't have good enough willpower.*'

Even if you complete a diet and feel like it's worked for you, the likelihood is you will be hooked on chasing numbers. You may still want to lose more. You may still want to tweak a little here and there – maybe just lose another 5lbs. You may still look in the mirror and find ways to pick your image apart.

The diet industry has us chasing a mirage that doesn't exist. It makes us believe that happiness is what we see in the mirror or a number on the scales.

> **Only when we realize that happiness
> is an inside job will we be able to
> ditch the diet mentality forever.**

When I used to starve myself to reach my '*goal weight*', I would get to that number on the scales at any cost. You name it I did it. When I got there – after weeks of not eating, liquid diets, caffeine overloading and working out like a maniac – guess what? Still not happy.

I would look in the mirror or step on the scales and say to myself, '*I need to just lose another 5lbs. Or, maybe 10 to be safe. Then I'll be good. Then I'll be perfect. Just a little bit more.*'

I look back at photos of me from this time and I was alarmingly thin. I had dieted like crazy, under the illusion that once I got to my goal weight I would suddenly feel comfortable in my skin.

But the goal weight wasn't the answer. I still wore baggy clothes to hide my body. I still didn't have the confidence to do those things I wanted to do. I still scrutinized photos of myself. And I still hated the idea of having to wear a swimsuit in public. *But if I just lost another 5 or 10lbs – then I'm sure I would be fine.*

Happiness is not a number or dress size.

I've worked with models that are considered by many women to have 'the perfect body' – and yet even these girls aren't happy. *Even these girls* are comparing themselves to other girls around them, agonizing over their food choices or wishing they had smaller waists, a bigger butt, a six-pack, etc. These girls are quite literally *stunning humans* and are being paid a small fortune to advertise clothing and products for big designer brands.

Similarly, I've worked with female bodybuilders and athletes who have dieted and trained non-stop in the lead-up for a physique competition and are admired by many aspiring fitness fanatics. Yet, backstage, these women are *still* scrutinizing themselves, wishing they had been just a little stricter, had a more ripped six-pack, more defined glutes, comparing themselves to all the other women in the competition, scrutinizing the photos – and then going home to massive binges.

To the audience they may have *the perfect physique* but are these women (and thousands of men, who are also affected by diet culture and the quest for the perfect body) truly happy, after they have dieted, strived for perfection, gone to extreme lengths?

After all – isn't happiness what we all *want?*

If we aren't striving to be happy, what are we doing?

The path to happy isn't in the diet.

It's not in the rules or the safe feeling of being 'in control'.

We are looking in all the wrong places for happiness.

What you're really chasing – what we're all really chasing – is to feel comfortable and happy in our own skin. The answer to this lies in your relationship with yourself.

Your relationship with food.

Your relationship with your body.

Everything else in your life is just a reflection of the most important relationship of your life – the one you have with YOU.

Goddess Shelley

'I've noticed that the more goodness I eat, the more my skin glows and I don't have that worried, angry look on my face any more. I look at food and instantly know whether my body would benefit from it or not.'

I had severe postnatal depression after my daughter was born. I was a young, single mum and food was my comfort. The problem was it came with strict rules. I could eat anything I wanted, as long as it didn't go over 1,200 calories a day.

Straight after giving birth I looked like a skeleton. I knew it wasn't right, but I somehow felt very proud that I could pull on my normal clothes four days after giving birth. Pretty soon my whole life turned around exercise and food, and I'd get angry if I hadn't been to the gym or had eaten over my calorie quota. Unwittingly I'd become trapped in a life I didn't want, but couldn't see any way out so I carried on.

Thanks to Mel, I've found a new positive mind-set and escaped. I've stopped calorie counting and only exercise when my body needs it, yet I am the happiest and healthiest I have ever been!

I can't believe how much has changed now... I have a life! A real life! One where I can relax in my own skin, and my mind is more positive, focused and happy! I enjoy every day, I listen to my body and I follow my inner rhythm, it's incredible!

What You're Really Chasing

'Feeling good is the primary intention.'
DANIELLE LAPORTE

When we chase a body. When we chase a goal weight. A dress size. A physique. It's not the body itself we truly desire. It is the feeling.

We so badly want to feel comfortable inside our own bodies, to feel good about ourselves, we chase the feeling we think this body will bring. The feeling we think this number or dress size will bring.

It's the same with material things – cars, money, houses, clothes – you name it. We don't want the things. We want the feeling we tell ourselves we will feel about ourselves when we have the things: accomplishment, achievement, success. To feel connected. Loved. Accepted. Whole. Satisfied.

If you never achieved the body or goal weight you were chasing, would you still be able to find happiness in yourself?

What if you actually arrived at your 'dream body' from doing a diet – but the happiness, feeling of wholeness and contentment never arrived with it?

Could you be happy in the here and now?

Could you love and respect your body where she is right now?

Could you work *with* her rather than against her? Make good choices to support a vision for good health driven by how you want to feel rather than how you want to look?

You cannot punish your body into a shape or size. You cannot hate your body into the body you want her to be. If you do, you will be fighting a losing battle for a very long time (*see the rest of your life*).

The only way is with love, respect, communication and patience.

> **You win the battle forever when you drop the weapon and refuse to attack or even partake in the fight.**
>
> **Food is not your enemy.**
>
> **Food is a team player.**
>
> **It wants to nourish your body, to support your life.**

The Raw Organic Vegan Paleo Sugar-free Gluten-free Macro 'Lifestyle'

Cut out meat.

Cut out dairy.

Cut out cooked foods.

Cut out sugar – *after convincing yourself you're addicted to it.*

Eat all organic.

Fast 'til 3 p.m.

Don't eat carbs after 4 p.m.

Cut out caffeine – *wait, no, add caffeine in as it raises your metabolism.*

Eat veg – *but don't eat starchy veg as it counts as carbohydrate.*

Eat protein – *but don't eat meat because it's bad for your health.*

Eat raw – *cooking foods destroys all the nutrition.*

Eat dairy for your main source of calcium – *but don't eat dairy because it's pumped full of hormones and antibiotics.*

Eat nuts – *but not too many. It's good fat, but fat is still fat. How many nuts is too many nuts?*

Don't eat sugar – *except natural sugar. Natural sugar's good for you, right? Scrap that... Don't eat natural sugar because at the end of the day it's still sugar so it's bad for you and will make you gain weight.*

Eat fruit because it's so good for you – *but not too much because it's carbohydrate and sugar, after all. All sugar is evil.*

Eat grains – *but don't eat grains because humans aren't supposed to eat grains.*

Eat high-carb, low-fat – *but also eat high-fat because your body needs fat and fatty acids are really beneficial for your heart health... but not too much...*

Follow the Paleo diet – *my friend Suzy knows someone who got down to 11 per cent body fat by doing that.*

On the other hand, if you choose vegan, you're bound to get thin. All vegans are thin... *But wait, I just read this article online that says vegans don't get enough protein?*

Overwhelmed, much? If you weren't then, you are now.

Maybe you've tried all the above. Maybe you went raw or cut out sugar or quit dairy and gluten or tried out the Paleo diet or vegan. Maybe you've researched all of the above and have become completely and utterly overwhelmed so haven't even attempted a single one because the very thought makes you want to scoff cookies and ice cream in secret.

A common theme with all of these diets is that they give you a set of rules to follow – which looks a lot like this:

1. Eat ABC.

2. Don't eat XYZ.

Sounds straightforward enough, right?

If only it was. Whichever diet you choose, you have to follow a set of rules that subconsciously you'll want to break free from.

Don't follow the crowd. Choose not to diet. Choose the anti-diet. Choose to live rule-free.

You will be fine.

Life is not supposed to stay in the lines.

Freedom is calling your name.

Goddess Grace

'I eat really healthily but I never deny myself anything that I really want. It feels good to be able to go out with my loved ones and enjoy spending time with them, and not think constantly about what I am eating.'

I would say that my food problems started due to health anxiety and I tried to make myself as healthy as possible by eating a 'perfect' diet – which for me meant only fruit and veg. I wasn't so concerned with losing weight – I just wanted to be healthy. But when the pounds started falling off, I was secretly pleased and kept trying to lose more, until I only weighed 5st 7lbs.

Now I realize how strange it was, but I liked being able to see my ribs and losing weight became an obsession too. I dreaded going on the scales in case I had put on any weight, and would vow to start a new diet if I did. I knew my family was terribly worried about me, I'd stopped menstruating and the doctors told me I was seriously jeopardizing my health.

Since working with Mel, I've learned to enjoy food again and nourish my body properly. I've gained weight and love eating a variety of different foods that weren't 'allowed' before.

I still feel insecure at times and I have a lot of regrets about the wasted energy I put into dieting, but in general I feel a lot better about myself and have started focusing on my dreams again. The beauty on the inside, rather than out.

When you 'screw up', skip a
workout or order a pizza,
it doesn't make you a bad
person. It makes you human.
Welcome to the club. There's
like seven billion of us.

The Answer Will Never Be in a Pill, Shake, Sachet or Tea

That includes skinny detox teas, herbal pills, caffeine pills that 'increase your metabolism and help you burn fat', diet or fat loss pills, meal-replacement shakes, supplements and herbal extracts from the top of a mountain that will help you 'drop a dress size in a week'…

All of the above.

Large numbers of corporations are vying for your money – the weight-loss and diet industry has specific and targeted ways to make money from your pain, your guilt, and your broken relationship with food and your body.

Social media accounts are paid vast amounts of money to share photos of themselves holding the latest fad diet tea, a detox drink, a protein shake, so more poor desperate dieters buy that product and cling to it for dear life.

Make no mistake – these companies know exactly what they are doing.

They trust you are desperately looking for something to cling to, instead of looking inwards, which of course you are.

*Dear Diet, it's not me, it's you.
I just don't think it's going
to work between us. You're
boring, you make me feel like
crap and I can't stop fantasizing
about cheating on you.*

The Problem with Cheat Meals

A 'cheat meal' or 'cheat day' is typically when someone is following a diet or is doing what they interpret to be their version of 'clean eating' throughout the week – then on Sunday or Friday night – or at any given point that they decide – they have a cheat meal. Usually planned out, this is basically a meal where you get a free pass to eat whatever the hell you want – and usually it's a shitload of junk.

Some people stop there. Others decide they deserve a full cheat *day* rather than just one meal. So they get a free pass for the whole of Sunday, or some will even give themselves a 90-minute window to binge on crap and then they go back to their 'clean eating' diet. Disordered eating having a field day.

Now, these cheat meals or days can get pretty horrific – they can get really gross. I have seen people having pizza, ice cream, takeaway and Oreos, and sometimes an entire table full of junk food that could feed four people, and they are having all of this as one meal. Yes – *all of the above in one sitting*. Cheat meals are not a joke, people. We can really go to extremes with it. And guess what? I fell into this pattern myself, too!

I used to eat chicken and broccoli for every meal throughout the week, plain salads and just boring meals – *really boring 'diet food'*. And then on Sunday, I would have a cheat meal, which was usually my free pass to get a takeaway, with a tub of ice cream afterwards. And I wouldn't just order one meal from a takeaway, I would order two or three and really go for it! Just so I felt like I'd really 'done it', so that then I could go back to my virtuous diet the next day.

This is a very popular trend in the fitness industry, especially bodybuilding. I hear a lot of people saying things like 'It's good for your body to have a shock by giving it some junk food now and again, so that you don't feel like you're depriving yourself!'

I don't think this is OK at all.

This cheat meal mentality means you are encouraging yourself to *look forward* to having a massive binge on junk food. And when you're eating a cheat meal, or just scheduling a cheat meal in, think about the message that you're sending to your body.

You're basically training your body to get excited about junk food. You're training your body to look forward to crap!

Just struggle now, just struggle with this diet, and then you're allowed the junk food. The junk food becomes glorified – it becomes a treat.

But it's not a treat at all really. It's not a treat for anyone, not least for your body.

Instead, create a happy, flexible lifestyle that you're so in love with, you never feel the urge to 'cheat' on it.

When you actually quit dieting, start nourishing your body and truly connecting and listening to it, then you won't want the junk food any more. I mean it.

And this is something that so many women have, at some point, said to me; 'I'm suddenly looking at the junk food I used to love, and now it makes me feel sick! I can't believe I used to look forward to putting this food in my body... the sight of it turns my stomach now.'

> **When you start to truly connect with what your body wants, you realize that it is not the crap she wants at all.**

Don't get me wrong. I definitely believe in a little bit of what you fancy, even if it's not so nutritious on paper. But when you fill your life with an abundance of great, healthy, real food – the stuff that you fancy *changes*, it really genuinely does.

Suddenly, you don't fancy the processed stuff so much or the sugar. If I eat something like a processed cereal bar now, it just tastes like sugary crap that I don't want inside my body – when a few years ago, I would have eaten two or three a day and thought nothing of it.

I'm a big advocate of having a 'treat' now and again. But have it when you actually *want* it – rather than scheduling in cheat meals or days when you will undoubtedly binge and go hell for leather, because you've been building up the anticipation for it. Trust me, you will feel so much happier and more at peace with your food when you live this way.

People ask me questions like *'Mel, do you never eat anything that's bad for you any more?'* Yeah, I do! Of course I do! I eat what I want to eat. Usually my body wants real food, the good stuff. But sometimes, I drink champagne all night and don't blink twice about eating a cupcake or ordering dessert at my favourite restaurant. Whatever food choice I make for my body, I take ownership over that choice, I commit to enjoying it, with no shame and no guilt, and I will get over it straight away and carry on living my life.

Saving yourself for a cheat meal will worsen your relationship with food, no doubt about it. All you're doing is training your body to look forward to junk food, which is not a lifestyle that will serve your body, ever.

What you'll soon start craving will be real, good, honest food. Food that your body agrees with you about. Foods that will serve you and make you feel good. You will also want to stop eating when your appetite is satiated because you'll know you won't feel good from carrying on past 'full' and into 'gross'.

Your primary intention is to feel good. Make choices to support that intention.

Goddess Caroline

'You wouldn't not service your car or your boiler so why not the one thing you own for your entire life, your body!'

I joined a slimming club just after my fiancé split up with me. At the time I thought the breakup was due to my 4st weight gain but it turned out he was having an affair… I stayed with the club for the next seven years and, in between the big loss and the gains back, lost a total of… 1st! The weekly weighs-in made me feel like a failure and led me to start bingeing. I would be strict all week and then blow out on weigh-in night because that didn't count, right?

Then I would feel awful. Sluggish, fat, sick, but it was OK because tomorrow I was back on the diet! Mental!

At precisely the same point that I began to realize that DIETS DON'T WORK, Mel appeared on my Facebook feed and her entire message confirmed what I had just discovered! Crazy huh... or maybe the universe pointed me in the right direction to help me out.

Being part of the Goddess Revolution has changed everything for me. I now love me and love my body. I have more love for my close friends and family, mostly because I am not obsessed about how I look to them and have stopped trying to impress them all the time. I have a newfound confidence, discovered spiritual wellbeing and, finally, got out of a destructive relationship (the first since the ex-fiancé) and started dating again!

Being free of the diet/binge cycle is so liberating, and I'm able to enjoy food again and own my choices. I now prefer to nourish my body with healthy foods because I love her. Yes, she is holding extra weight and is clumsy at times but she is all mine and, in turn, this has given me so much confidence. I used to live by 'fake it till you make it' and pretend I was confident, but now I really am!

. . . .

When we diet, we spend so
much energy focused on
what we are losing, rather
than what we are gaining.
It's a negative way of
thinking from the get-go.

Diets Tell You NO

Diets make you constantly *deny* yourself. All the emphasis is placed on what you are in *denial* of. It's no wonder they make us miserable.

It's all cut out sugar, cut out dairy, cut out wheat, cut out gluten, cut out carbs, cut out meat, cut out coffee, cut out alcohol… It's little wonder we fold and wind up feeling completely useless for not sticking to it – it's all focused on **loss** and not focused on gain.

Instead, I challenge you to focus on all the wonderful foods you should be increasing instead!

When we diet we feel somewhat like we are living a **lesser life** because we are depriving ourselves. But what if we focused on what we were gaining and started including what's missing instead? Our lives would feel fuller, richer, happier, and we would feel better than ever!

Stop counting calories and stop weighing yourself, and just notice how you start to feel differently.

The most important thing you can ever do for your body is to stop scrutinizing her in the mirror every day. Literally, just stop doing it. **Start focusing on how your body FEELS.** Rather than how she looks.

What foods make her feel amazing? What increases your energy, rather than depletes it?

Again, it's a case of connecting and listening to your body. It may be hard at first – but you have a lifetime of practice ahead of you, and likely a lot of years making up for all the ignoring you've done 'til now.

But wait... will I still lose weight?

I hear you control freaks panicking – I hear you!

If I stop my dieting and restricting and start listening to my body... I'm bound to gain weight, right?

Wrong. If you truly listen to what your body wants, cook meals using real foods that your body craves and listen to your body to stop when you're full – your weight **will** come to find its natural balance. You **will** start to feel more connected than ever. You **will** start to feel happier than ever in your body. Your body wants you to have a balanced, 'normal' relationship with food. She doesn't like being starved one week and stuffed the next. It's abuse.

If you follow the principles in this book – you will live a richer, happier and more fulfilled life around food and your body. If you're carrying excess weight due to overeating, bingeing or emotional eating – you will begin to lose it quite effortlessly, without any need to control it whatsoever.

If you have a history of starving yourself – eating a very restricted number of calories every day and are underweight – and **now** start listening to your body then, yes, there's a good chance you will gain some of the weight you lost from drastic dieting. Your body will find its natural balance where it belongs – in prime healthy condition. Not underweight and not overweight. Your body wants to support your *life*, in the unique chapter and path that you are currently on.

This is NOT a weight-loss plan.

This is a way to completely rebuild your relationship with food and your body for life. This is a way to live free from the shackles of the dieting world (*take the shackles off my feet so I can dance!*) and truly step into the Goddess you were born to be.

Part III

Tearing Up the Rulebook

Refuse to follow the crowd.

Refuse to conform to the rules.

Rules are made to be broken.

Break them with great delight.

*Live a life without rules
or restrictions.*

*Join the revolution – stop
hating your body.*

*Stop trying to 'fix'
yourself with diets.*

Pay attention and listen.

Live a life of freedom.

The Goddess Manifesto

- I connect with my body on a daily basis.
- I allow myself to feel my feelings, rather than trying to eat them.
- I show my body love by respecting her.
- I enjoy eating real, whole foods in abundance.
- I do not allow myself to feel guilty about food.
- I forgive myself for not being perfect and embrace my imperfections with love.
- I enjoy socializing and eating out with friends.
- I count nutrients and colours on my plate, never calories or grams.
- I adore time in my kitchen.
- I prioritize making time for myself.
- I never abuse or project hate onto my body.
- I do not allow myself to be controlled by the scales or a tape measure or a dress size.

- ❧ I am grateful for my body and what she is capable of.

- ❧ I eat mindfully and when I am hungry.

- ❧ I only do exercise that I enjoy!

- ❧ I allow myself to be playful, try new things and be adventurous.

- ❧ I understand that to get the body I want, I must start my loving and respecting the body I have.

What Kind of a Relationship Are You In?

If your relationship with food were a romantic relationship, what kind of a relationship would you be in? How would it look? How would it feel? (And would your girlfriends approve or tell you to stop calling him and delete his number?)

Would it be a loving, caring, two-sided relationship?

A relationship fuelled by infatuation, greed and pleasure?

An intense, controlling relationship, with rules and feelings of imprisonment?

An abusive relationship?

Would it be a highly addictive relationship – one that you *know* is bad for you – all your friends tell you it's bad for you – but you keep coming back for more? (*We've all dated that person!*)

Or would it be a boring, monotonous relationship with no adventure or change from the ordinary?

Would it be a stale, regimented relationship during the week, followed by naughty, indulgent flings on the weekends?

Ooh… such a good question, right? Really makes you think…

When I reflect on my past relationship with food and my body, I was for *sure* in an abusive relationship. I stayed in it for years and continued to fuel it by repeating the same addictive patterns.

But through healing, self-love and learning how to nurture that oh-so-important relationship, it has blossomed into something beautiful – with a gorgeous balance of fun, excitement and freedom, grounded by a deep sense of loyalty and true friendship.

It's so important to remember this too, Goddess:

You're already IN the most important relationship of your life. Your relationship with YOU.

Your relationship with FOOD is a huge contributor to that relationship. It's about **you**. It's about **your self-worth**.

When your relationship with food takes an upgrade, so does your relationship with yourself. So does your **self-worth**. And when your self-worth takes an upgrade, so does every other area of your life.

When you have a beautiful relationship with **you**, you become a **magnet** for beautiful relationships in your life – friendships, romantic relationships, family. Food is a great place to start, Goddess. It's oh-**so**-important to look at the bigger picture here.

'I wish I had spent more time counting calories'
…said no one ever.

Stop Tracking, Start Living

Counting or tracking calories is an extremely out-dated way to approach your lifestyle and can be incredibly damaging to your relationship with food. It is a complete myth that all calories are created equal.

I saw a graphic on social media recently that really drove me up the wall. Someone had drawn two pictures and put them side by side – a big greasy cheeseburger on one side and a superfood salad, topped with avocado, walnuts, butternut squash, feta, quinoa and pumpkin seeds on the other. All this great, nutritious green food sitting opposite this big, greasy burger. The calories were underneath and to my surprise – and no doubt a lot of other people's too – they equated to the same number of calories.

People were then leaving comments like, 'Well, may as well just keep eating my Big Macs!' 'See – no point in eating salads after all!'

No, no, no, no, NO! Can you hear how *wrong* that is? *Common sense* tells us that these two meals could not be further apart.

The diet industry, and to some extent the medical profession, has done this to us. It has taught us to live by calories in, calories out. Use the system and you can't go wrong.

If we eat a Big Mac with 500 calories, we'd better make sure we burn 500 calories on the treadmill at the end of the day, and then it's like it never happened! Right?

Wrong.

You don't need me to tell you this because you're a smart human, but the nutrition in that burger is, of course, next to zero. The ingredients used to create and preserve that burger are things I wouldn't feed to my pets, my worst enemy, let alone my own body.

If one person ate a cheeseburger every day for the rest of her life and one person ate a superfood salad every day for the rest of her life, who do you think would be healthier? Who would lose weight and who would gain it? Who would *live longer?*

Yet so many of us are still holding on to the calories approach, thinking that they matter and, perhaps, tracking them relentlessly with apps – which only keeps us trapped in a world of judgement, restriction and punishment. If you eat 800 calories a day and that consists of a croissant and a chocolate bar, do you think you are going to have a healthy, lean body in the long run? How do you think your body is going to feel?

I used to try my best to stick to 1,000 calories a day, sometimes fewer. I would hit the gym every day and not leave 'til I had burned exactly 1,000 calories. The tracking life is *grim*, people.

Did I lose weight doing this? Barely. But I sure as hell became completely obsessed with numbers! I was constantly miserable, snapped at my loved ones, had no fun whatsoever and avoided social occasions because I cared so much about sticking to my calorie intake and outtake. Grim, grim, grim.

Why count calories when you could be being more present in your relationships, living your ideal life, following your dreams and nourishing your body with real foods?

If you're reading this and you're somebody who obsessively counts calories – I sincerely hope you're starting to rethink your strategy.

> **The real honest food, what our body
> truly craves, doesn't come with
> a calorie label or numbers.**

I know it sounds like a hard challenge but stopping the constant counting will give you so much more freedom and fun in your life around food. I know what you want right now is just to hit those numbers – but what you truly desire deep down is to be happy and free in your body. What you truly desire is to feel happy, to feel comfortable in your own skin, to be accepted by yourself. Set yourself free from the numbers game. You will never win at it.

Break Up with Your Scales, Too

You probably saw this one coming. Your scales. They have to go.

So many of us are hopping on the scales every Monday or even every morning, and waiting to be answered, 'Are you a good person today or a bad person today?' 'How are you allowed to feel today – will it be virtuous or will it be worthless?' We ask a piece of glass or plastic for validation, and then let it run our day and dictate our food choices.

Why? Why do we try to validate ourselves with a number on the scales?

That number doesn't tell you how smart you are, how aligned you are in your life choices, how good your ethics and morals are, what a kind person you are, how beautiful you are, how fit or strong you are, how generous and loving you are... So why are we so hooked on this number?

What is it actually telling us? Our effect on gravity!

It doesn't even tell us if we are gaining muscle and losing fat. It just tells us how heavy we are.

And here's another thing – if you're exercising using weights, your body will be changing. You're likely to *look* slimmer but weigh heavier. All the scales know is a number dictated by gravity.

This is possibly *the single* most important thing you absolutely have to do in order to welcome in a happy relationship with food and your body – **break up with your scales.** Recognize that it is a toxic relationship that always leaves you feeling bad.

Trust me, I feel you, I've been there. I know it's hard and you want to skip this part and pretend you don't have to do this. But there's just no way around this one. If you are struggling to love your body, struggling to find that healthy lifestyle you know is waiting for you, and you are still weighing yourself compulsively, then you are taking one step forwards and two steps back.

You are asking to be validated by a piece of plastic or metal or glass.

Even if you think the scales don't impact your happiness, chances are, they do. Because they are making you compare yourself to the number you had a year ago, five years ago, two weeks ago or yesterday morning.

And guess what. We are moving **forwards**, people, not back! If you keep comparing yourself *now* to your old self, before you had a baby, when you were at college or when you were on that beach holiday, do you *see* how much that is holding you back from stepping into the life you want? If you're constantly looking *backwards* and not forwards?

You're in a brand new chapter now, Goddess, away from dieting, away from misery. You are creating a beautiful abundant lifestyle with no rules. How happy do you want to feel?

So, if I haven't made it clear enough:

BREAK UP WITH YOUR SCALES!

If you aren't brave enough to throw them out in the trash, just take out the battery and chuck that away. Or, if you really do need even more baby steps, just get someone to hide them somewhere so you can't find them. Or put them in a different room, somewhere you never go. Or, put them in a box and then put the box somewhere you can't reach. But mainly, just freaking do it! Just get rid of them and break that habit however which way you can.

Important Aside

If your medical practitioner has told you that you must weigh yourself for medical reasons, then do not ignore them, but please – only a maximum of once every few weeks. I want us to do some real work on your self-worth and make some huge shifts together. Consistently weighing yourself at the same time will do nothing but leave you stuck. You will know from reading this chapter whether you have a dependency on scales or not. If you want this to work, you must above all be honest with yourself.

It's also *so* important to realize that your weight fluctuates day to day, hour to hour even, depending on your stress levels, water intake, how much you've sweated, your digestion, your time of the month, your exercise of choice… so it's really *not* a good idea to keep checking on that number.

The best way to track your progress is just to notice how you *feel* in your body and in your clothes. And notice how your body feels when you wake up and get out of bed first thing in the morning.

*Goal weight – sexy as f*ck!*

The Art of Abundance

'What is called genius is the abundance of life and health.'

HENRY DAVID THOREAU

Conquering the battles inside your head promoting restriction and rules, starts with allowing the love to flood in – in total, unrestricted abundance. Making friends with yourself and treating you as a number-one priority, instead of living in a constant state of attack.

This is the new mind-set that absolutely changed my life – and one that you have to commit to in order to be happy in your body… AND nourish yourself without deprivation.

Start cultivating a mind-set that says abundance, abundance, abundance.

Anything is possible. You can create anything with the power of your mind. And a huge part of this shift is embracing the fact that any food is available for you to eat. No food is metaphorically off the table. No food is out of bounds. No food is 'bad' or 'evil' or 'on the naughty list'. No food choice means you 'failed'. There is no pass or fail. There is no good or bad.

That might sound like a scary concept. I know it was for me. I had tremendous fears around certain foods that would 'trigger' me, make me binge eat or that I had just sworn to myself I would never eat because they were such 'bad' foods.

There are probably quite a few foods that you have on the safe list or the unsafe list. You may have been swearing yourself off big food groups too, such as anything that remotely feels like a 'carb'. I invite you to put all this aside: all the rules that you've been telling yourself around food or justified you not eating certain things. And I invite you to take your rules and say loud and clear to yourself, 'Screw them!'

You heard me. Screw all of them. Throw them up in the air. Among all of the other reasons listed in this book to screw the rules – life is simply too short to imprison yourself with them. Following rules means you'll always be encouraging a relationship with food that feels trapped and unexpressed.

I can hear you thinking… *If I let go of all my rules and eat in abundance, won't I binge eat and gain a ton of weight?*

When I say abundance I do not mean stuff your gorgeous face silly. I do not mean binge. I mean – release the rules and be civil again with all those fear foods, instead of living in fear of them.

It's the difference between holding on to hatred and grudges with an old friend who hurt you, *or* agreeing to see past your differences and acknowledging them in the room instead of scowling.

Embrace the fact that all food is now readily available to you – in abundance – and you have the power to take it or leave it, in exactly the way your body wants to be nourished. Even the foods you may have created a story about – the ones you think make you gain weight just by looking at them, for example. When you stop living in fear of these foods and acknowledge that you have the simple choice to take it or leave it in that moment – because it's *your body, your rules* – you take back your power day by day and stop feeling like food is running your life.

Choose how you nourish your body

When you start eating with a sense of mindfulness and respect for food and your body – when you really start communicating with your body, talking, and listening – you should eventually be able to identify when you're hungry and when you're full.

For many of us this entire idea of abundance is undoing a lifetime of bad habits and patterns – but it is 100 per cent possible for you – and it is a practice that will serve you for life.

I invite you to eat all the foods that make your body *feel good* and reject the foods that you *know* make your body feel rubbish.

Now, there's a big difference between food making your body feel good – and the taste of a food pleasuring your mouth for a few seconds. Really start to listen to what foods make your **body** feel exactly the way you want it to feel, and what foods really don't make your body feel good at all.

Screw the rules. Your body wants freedom.

Dieting Is a Full-time Job

When I think back to my dieting days, I am saddened by how much energy and time it sucked out of my life. It was like having a full-time job – except nobody was paying me and I was working overtime for a boss I could never please.

When I wasn't feeling bad about the last meal I ate, I was thinking about what I was going to eat next. If I wasn't thinking about that, I was thinking about the next diet I was going to start. If I wasn't thinking about that, I was thinking about which exercise class I had to revolve my day around. And when I wasn't thinking about that, I was thinking about the number that the scales had told me that day and calculating how quickly I could lose x amount of weight before a certain date. When I wasn't thinking about that, I was thinking about how many calories I had eaten that day. And, when I wasn't thinking about calories, I was wondering if the person I was with thought I looked fat. When I wasn't doing that, I was regretting the choice of outfit I'd made, fretting about whether my legs looked too big in those jeans, if my muffin top made me feel sick, or if my arms looked fat in that photo.

Wow. Not a lot of room for a life in there.

I must have neglected so many moments, missed so many opportunities, been completely distracted in relationships and friendships, social events and family gatherings – because of the time and energy I spent obsessing over food and my weight.

Dieting *is* a full-time job. Being a dieter takes a huge amount of time, energy and commitment. It's a rollercoaster, but it's a rollercoaster you can get off right now, and make the choice to reclaim your life again.

You (probably) already have a job.
Your life has a purpose.
Your life has meaning.
Your relationships have meaning.
Your friendships have meaning.
Reclaim your body.
Reclaim your life.
Make a start by reclaiming your relationship
with food and your body.

Goddess Theresa

'I still have days when self-doubt creeps in, and old habits rear their ugly head, but they're becoming fewer and far between. Free from the scales and the power they had over me, I no longer reach for junk food when emotional (or very rarely), and I am kind to myself.'

I was a fairly healthy active child, but that changed when I started secondary school and was bullied – not just for my weight but my appearance too. At sixth form I was at my biggest and miserable, and so the diets began. I would binge at weekends, hating myself, then promise myself I would start again next week. Then would eat as little as possible for as long as possible, until I couldn't hold out any longer and the binge cycle would begin again.

I finally managed to get my weight back into healthy range, just before I got married. But I knew it was due to crazy dieting and I was FAR from healthy. Emotionally I was still the fat teenager. I may have been a healthy weight but inside I still felt like a failure – and dieting was my new safety net. Looking back I realized that I was quite hard to live with too – going out was a huge deal and it would take me hours to choose what to wear, I would never put myself forward for jobs I wanted because I felt so useless and I would constantly put myself down and end up in tears.

OK, I still have a long way to go, but since joining the Goddess Revolution I'm a much happier version of me. My whole family has noticed, particularly my children, and my husband has been totally supportive. I haven't weighed myself in months and I'm not consumed by thoughts of numbers. I make time for me and, day by day, my mind-set is changing – and that's huge.

I have made peace with my past – I've forgiven myself for the way I treated my body – and am excited by life! I took the leap, got out of my comfort zone and am now a qualified PiYo instructor – I would never done this without Mel and the Goddesses behind me!

A good friend texted me after my daughter's party and said, 'Today I saw you, you looked so happy, so slim, so fit, so happy!' And a lady who attends my PiYo class said, 'You are so confident and energetic, I wish I could be more like you' – if only she had known me a year ago!

. . . .

The Future You

When I say 'Future You', I mean the dreamy version of you – the one you sometimes daydream about and wistfully think, *some day*. The one where you are so happy and content in your body, you love your body so much, and you are living this gorgeous healthy lifestyle that just feels effortless to you.

This is the version of you that you perhaps picture and imagine every time you start a new diet. Maybe it's an old version of you, in which case we are going to rewrite it. As I said earlier, if you're constantly trying to get *back* to an old version of you – your old body, when you were younger, when you were happier, when you were healthier – you're going backwards. Aka, the wrong way, Goddess.

You are in a completely different place now than you were back then, and you want be going forwards: moving into a *new* chapter, a *new* you, the dream you, the future you. And, of course, we will be stepping into her right now – not waiting to be 'ready' or wait for a certain number or dress size.

So, what does the Future You look like? How does she feel? And what are you waiting for? Visualize it.

* What does a day look like for the Future You?

* If you had all the time, and all the money – how would you spend your day?

* What would you do for your body each day, or each week?

My Future Me wakes up early and does some yoga and meditation to start the day. Then I make a big breakfast of a green smoothie, maybe eggs or pancakes. Then I catch up with my emails and check in with my Goddesses online and run my Academy from my laptop. I write blogs and content, and create recipes, and then maybe I go for a swim or a long walk outside. Finally in the evening I eat out with a friend or loved one and enjoy delicious healthy food. Or maybe I cook for myself at home.

In my ideal day you can see there are things that I associate with my body – health and vitality are both important to me, and they're obviously important to you too! So, what does a day in the life of the Future You look like, and what are you doing every day to nourish your body during that day?

What foods are you eating? What are you drinking? What exercise are you doing, and what are your reasons for doing it?

In your ideal day, I suspect you're not spending the whole day fretting about staying under 1,200 calories, you aren't weighing yourself every morning (because you know that doesn't make you happy) and you aren't taking photos of yourself in the mirror either. You'll also notice that you are simply moving your body because it feels good, not because you want to burn calories. It's just part of your lifestyle, because it makes you happy and alive in your body. Right?

Pick one or two things out of the Future You, and start bringing them into your present life.

For example, if the Future You goes to a dance class every day because you love it, then start going to a dance class once a week, or even once a fortnight, right now.

If your Future You has a personal trainer but right now you can't afford one, then maybe just book in for a one-off session once a month?

If your ideal day includes 10 minutes of meditation every morning, but right now you can't find the time to do that, then start doing just 10 minutes every Sunday instead.

It doesn't mean doing everything, every day straight off, it just means getting into the **feeling** of how it is to have these things be a part of your life. You deserve to have these things right now, even if it is just in a smaller way.

You might be asking, 'What on earth has this got to do with me losing weight and getting the body I want?'

Well, more than you think, Goddess. If your life doesn't have any sense of feeling like the life you really want – and not making you happy – then this could be *the* very cause of your overeating, your mindless eating patterns or the reason you keep self-sabotaging when you try to eat well. It might not be that your life sucks because of your food issues, but that your food issues are a direct result of *your life sucking.* Please don't take offence. If you aren't *enjoying* your life and all the things in it, then it's little wonder that you're turning to food to feel in control or numb the feelings of discontentment.

If in doubt, visit the Future You. Ask her, 'What will you thank me for doing? What will you thank me for getting rid of?'

Visit your Future You often and ask her for advice. She might be six months down the line, a year down the line or five years down. What would she have you do? How can you honour the Future You right now?

To have the body you love,
you must start by loving
the body you have.

Your Dream Body

When I say your dream body, what initially comes up for you? Maybe you *think* your dream body is the one belonging to that model you follow on Instagram with the crazy tight abs and the perfect butt? Maybe you *think* it's the body of a celebrity, or the body you had when you were 20?

Well, if you are chasing any of the above as *your* dream body – and especially if you're chasing it with thoughts of hate and punishment towards your own body – I can quite confidently say that you are never going to be satisfied and you are never going to be happy.

Your dream body still has to be *your* body. Forgive me for pointing out the obvious, but you cannot *swap* bodies with somebody else.

Even if you did all the same exercises as someone else and ate the exact same food every day as them too – your body would *still not morph into theirs.*

Your body is unique to you.
Respect that and work with her.

I want you to really rephrase what your dream body means to you. In this chapter, I want you to start thinking about where you're at in your life right now, and how your body can best support you.

When we talk about your dream body, rather than immediately focusing on how you want your body to *look*, I want you to start focusing on how you want your dream body to *feel*.

How do you think you will *feel* in this dream body? Light, agile, strong, empowered, fresh, healthy, feminine, alive?

If you've been on diets that have made you feel tired, hungry and weak and you've kidded yourself that as soon as it's over, *then* you'll be allowed to feel great, then I'm afraid you should realize right now, that is a one-way ticket to feeling very disappointed.

When you follow what truly makes your body **feel** the way you want it to feel and do things that consistently support, encourage and reinforce that feeling, **that** is when you are on the road to living your dream life and having your dream body. Then it feels exactly how you want it to **feel**.

You can have it ALL

How would you act if you had your dream body? If you were living your dream life? If you were at your perfect weight, right now?

What would the Future You be doing every day in this life?

You'd be making choices that feel wonderful to your body. You'd be exercising because it feels damn good. Saying no to the things you don't want. Not ever forcing anything that doesn't feel good. Living abundantly, freely and at total peace with yourself. Never feeling guilty around food.

Think about how great that feels. It can be yours, in an instant, if you decide to embody the feeling right now and live *that story* instead of your old one.

What's Your Why?

Start thinking about why it's so important to you *personally* that you make this shift. What is it that you really want? Be totally and completely honest.

Whatever your past struggles around food, weight or body image – what is it that's driving you to make a change?

What is your big why? What is making you want to end this struggle?

It could be that you are looking to welcome love into your life and you know that's pretty hard to do if you don't love yourself first. Or maybe you're shedding old chapters of your life and are ready to step into a brand new one. It could be that your relationship is really suffering because of how you feel about yourself – I know mine did.

It might be that you've pushed your friends or your family away because you can't relax during social occasions, because all you're thinking about is the food and what you have made it mean. Or it could be that you and your partner are trying to get pregnant right now – and you know your body needs to be a safe and healthy environment, fuelled with love and good nutrition.

For me, as I described earlier, my main reason for wanting to end the battle with my body and cultivate a beautiful relationship with her was that I realized how desperately I wanted to be a mum one day but immediately started experiencing panic-stricken, fear-driven egocentric thoughts about conception, pregnancy and passing my bad eating habits and poor body image on to my children.

I decided in that very moment that enough was enough and the battle had to end immediately. This wasn't about me any more. This was about my future family.

That was my BIG WHY.

If this in any way resonates with you – know this.

Your children can't help but emulate you.

Even if you think you are *saying* all the right things to them, they will still copy Mummy and how you behave – around food, around people and how you speak to yourself in the mirror or when trying on clothes.

> *Take responsibility. Choose to be a role model to your children and the children that come after that. They may not follow your advice, but they will follow your example.*

When you find your why and your relationship with your food and your body takes an upgrade, so does every other area of your life. Suddenly you will find so much more joy in everything you do.

You will feel happy and wild and free again, and as if you can really take everything and anything you want out of life! And here's the magic – you really can!

Part IV

Get Full Up –
What Are You
Hungry For?

Say 'Yes!' to meals out, birthday celebrations, baby showers and hen dos, and thoroughly enjoy every moment of them. But remember, nobody (hopefully) is actually force-feeding you. You are, after all, the boss of your life, and indeed, your food choices.

You Can't Eat Your Feelings

When we think of hunger, we think of our bellies grumbling, asking to be fed. But I want to ask you, honestly, Goddess, *What is your soul hungry for?* What is it most in life that you are hungry for right now?

* Success?

* Intimacy?

* Purpose?

* Validation?

* Sensuality?

* Creativity?

* Acceptance?

* Freedom?

What do you most *desire?* What are you not getting from your life, your environment, your relationships that could be making you turn to overeating?

Hunger vs. Cravings

Start to pay attention to what your body is telling you – are you hungry or are you experiencing a craving or desire for *something other than food*?

If you've ever been on a diet then you might have thought it was a smart move to try and ignore your hunger – or try and push away your cravings by distracting them.

Instead of ignoring your cravings, hating them or trying to distract them, I ask you to start embracing them, respecting them and carefully observing them.

When you begin to do this, you will no longer be a slave to cravings. Cravings are here to tell you something. What do you most crave in life? What are you really craving now, if you take food out of the equation?

In life we all long to feel connected, accepted, whole, fulfilled. We yearn to feel loved and accepted, by others and by ourselves.

Your cravings are here to help guide
you towards your most authentic self,
and your most purpose-driven life.

There's a difference between emotional cravings and real hunger.

An emotional craving is a strong and sudden desire to eat food right now, which can also cause a sense of panic and urgency. If you sit with it for 10–15 minutes it *will* pass. You feel it in your head, not your stomach.

Real hunger comes on gradually over a period of hours in your stomach. It doesn't feel urgent. It doesn't cause you to panic. You actually have time to figure out what it is that will satisfy your body. But OH, we try to. When something difficult happens in our lives, we go into survival mode. Unfortunately we're not so great at understanding our real *feelings*. Most of us are taught from a young age to put a brave face on and soldier through. We likely have had years of practice of using food as comfort or as a reward.

What about listening to how you really feel?

When we are emotionally eating, essentially we are feeling something uncomfortable that we don't want to feel or don't understand, and then using food to try and *numb* those feelings. But numbing is, as you know, only temporary.

When we are emotionally eating, all we are really doing is trying to *drown out* feelings, or *push down* feelings. We are using food as a way to *opt out* of feeling these feelings.

Often, when we feel rejected, lonely or stressed, food becomes the thing we turn to immediately. Food feels comforting and loving. Food feels like love to us.

But what if you actually sat down with these feelings and asked yourself honestly what was going on? What if you actually stopped for a moment, got curious and asked, 'What am I really experiencing right now?'

Think about how normal it is to numb our feelings: to have a cup of coffee in the morning or a glass of wine in the evening to 'take the edge off' the day. Think about how socially acceptable it is to use food as a way to comfort yourself when you're down. Or perk you up when you need to be energized.

What are you trying to OPT OUT of feeling?
Newsflash: You can't eat your feelings!

Here's a really important tool that I hope you will take and use every time you want to dive deep into your relationship with food and heal negative patterns and unwanted habits.

Simply stop, slow down your breath and ask yourself, 'How am I feeling right now?' That's literally all it is. How am I feeling right now? And then answer with how you are feeling. Define your feeling. And then, instead of using food, *sit* with the feeling.

You have probably heard the term 'mindful eating' – which can feel like the hardest thing to do when you are used to turning to food to numb every feeling you experience. But mindful eating is also known as *paying attention*.

Stopping. Breathing. Paying attention and asking what's up with this – how am I feeling? Get curious. Observe your feelings. Become your own detective.

If there is one lesson you take from this entire book please let it be to pay attention to these feelings. You might not need to put your hand on your heart and close your eyes – maybe you just need to slow down and quietly question how you're feeling.

I'm challenging you to *catch yourself in the act*, right before you're called to eat, or even *mid-binge*. There will be a moment where you *know* you have the choice to stop and make a better choice for yourself, or carry on abusing yourself with food.

Having the power to stop yourself before a binge is pretty life-changing by itself.

I now tend to ask myself 'How am I feeling?' before every meal and every time I eat. Now, 95 per cent of the time, it's 'hungry'. But sometimes still, I find myself wanting to emotionally eat. Here's what happens when that occurs:

Q: 'How am I feeling?'

A: *'You're feeling overwhelmed and stressed.'*

Q: 'Is food the answer to overwhelm or stress?'

A: *'No. I would be eating the food with all the wrong intentions, the wrong energy surrounding the process, and in a stressed-out state' – which means I would probably inhale the whole damn thing.*

What *actually* calms my overwhelm down is self-care, yoga,

meditating or simply deep breathing, going for a walk, turning my phone off or getting off social media for a day, reading a book and writing.

Q: 'How am I feeling?'

A: 'Exhausted.'

Q: 'Is food the answer to exhaustion?'

A: 'No. Sleep is. Go take a power nap or crash early tonight. Food won't make you any less exhausted. Sleep is the answer here, not carbs.'

Easier said than done, I know. But it's all about practice. You're not gonna be like, tick, got the Goddess way *sussed – now what?* This is a principle and a tool you can live by for the rest of your life and practise every single day – and, yes, it takes time.

So how are you feeling, Goddess? Do any of the following emotions resonate with how you feel before you reach for food?

- Angry?
- Anxious?
- Stressed?
- Overwhelmed?
- Lonely?
- Bored?
- Lost?
- Disappointed?
- Exhausted?
- Upset?
- Excited?
- Happy?
- Panicked?
- Rejected?
- Disconnected?

It might be painful to go here, Goddess – but it's absolutely a vital part of your growth and healing process. Please – trust me and do this.

By being mindful and observing yourself – getting curious about your feelings and truly connecting and listening to your body – you send your body the message 'I'm here. I'm ready to listen. I'm ready to cooperate, instead of using food to mask or numb the feelings.' And Goddess – that message goes a long, long way.

Goddess Sally

'Sometimes, old habits begin to sneak back in, but I'm so totally aware of them now that I recognize them and am able to work out why they're rearing their heads and deal with them.'

I was at a complete loss with my eating habits. I felt continually frustrated and angry that I couldn't eat what (I thought) I wanted, and that if I did, I would put on weight. It felt it was SO unfair! How could other (slim) people eat what they wanted and not gain weight? I thought it must be my genes. I had tried EVERY diet going and found if I stuck to it, I could lose 10lbs in a week. If I didn't, I could put on 7lbs – and frequently did. I thought this was how I would spend my life, and didn't believe I would ever be slim for more than a few months at a time. I thought I would battle my emotional eating demons forever!

My food issues began when I was a child. When Dad was having a bad day, he would be physically and mentally violent, and my mum consoled us – me, my brother and herself – with food. Cake, chocolate, ice cream. It lessened the pain slightly for a little while, but as I got older, I continued to turn to food for comfort. When I was a teenager, my dad would feed me up on excessive amounts of my favourite foods and praise how much I ate, so I ate some more (praise from him was a rarity) and more and more. Then, when I put weight on, he would criticize me and tell people I was built like my mum, who he called obese and disgusting during arguments.

I thought that dieting was the only way to be thin – I had been well and truly brainwashed – and the only reason I was fat was because I couldn't stick to a diet! It didn't occur to me that by taking part in the whole circus I was setting myself up for a fall. I thought that I would be on a diet for the rest of my life. I really believed that that was the way life would be: I would lose weight, keep it off for a couple of months, pile it back on plus some more and then lose weight again.

Mel showed me step by step how to unpick my eating habits. Why I ate the way I did. Why I ate the things I did. Why I had the existing relationship that I had with food and my body. By understanding my behaviour and the reasons for it, I was able to let it all go!

I now eat to nourish my body and soul! Most of the time, I choose foods that give me energy and make me feel good. Now I'm 2st lighter and I eat what I actually want and I enjoy my food! Listening to my body, I've discovered that she really does know what she wants! If I eat something that's not so nourishing, that's OK too – I don't beat myself up and say horrible things to myself any more! But now I understand that it's no longer about the food, I have other ways of dealing with a bad day. I'll run a bath, have my nails done, meet up with my mum or friends, or buy myself something nice – anything that nourishes my soul.

. . . .

Quit the Distractions

When you're eating – eat.

That means stop eating on the go, while working at your desk, checking emails or scrolling through social media. In fact, don't look at your phone when you're eating. Focus solely on the food and the meal. This is the biggest mistake that we busy women love to make when it comes to food – we don't slow down and just eat. We try to multitask with food.

And, yes, I get that everyone is busy. But you *do* have time to eat. You absolutely have to start prioritizing your food and your wellbeing. They go hand in hand. Would you let your child or your employee eat the way you do? Constantly on the go, not having any rest, shovelling food down and grabbing it while running out the door?

You would say 'Whoa! Take a break. Eat your lunch in peace. Slow down.' Don't let it be any different for you. Eat without distractions, without running around, not on your commute – eat consciously, mindfully. Pay attention to your food.

What Fills You Up?

'Respond to every call that excites your spirit.'
RUMI

Pay attention and get curious!

* What in life makes you feel so full up, you could burst?

* What makes your heart flutter?

* What makes you feel complete, connected, whole?

* What is it that you're curious about?

* What deeply fascinates you?

* What is it that truly feeds you?

* What is it that truly nourishes your soul?

The answers to these questions are usually found in creative activities or pastimes that are uncomplicated and come easily to you, or things that make your eyes go wide with fascination and curiosity. Things that immediately make you smile or light you up.

It could be anything: writing, reading, painting, yoga, meditation, cooking, knitting, sewing, make-up, artwork, acting, singing, photography, dancing, playing a musical instrument, painting, designing, making jewellery, making candles – the possibilities are endless.

And don't think you have to pick just one! We put a lot of pressure on ourselves to find our true 'calling' in life – but the truth is, you probably have several. And you should absolutely dabble in all of them! Yep – permission to dabble is hereby granted!

Ask your inner child

If you're stuck and have no idea what fills you up, your inner child may know.

Go way back to when you were growing up. What filled you up then? What did you absolutely love to do and would have done all day long 'til the cows came home? What filled you up before you got stuck in 'adulting' and society told you that you should stop doing things just for fun and always attach an end goal or an outcome?

What nourished your soul when you were a child?

I was always a very creative, free-spirited child and would fill my time outside school with dancing, writing, reading and sports. Astrology and mermaids always fascinated me too. Growing up, I fancied myself as a ballerina, a novelist, a pop star, a mermaid, an artist, a magazine editor, a Spice Girl and everything in between.

What did your inner child absolutely love to do *just* for fun, before she grew into an adult with responsibilities and expectations of how she thought she *should* spend her time?

By nourishing your soul, you are far less likely to feel the need to fill up the void with food.

Maybe, just maybe, that void could be filled up with the sort of creativity and pure joy you enjoyed as a child – and that has been missing in your life since.

> *We do not stop playing because we grow old*
> *– we grow old because we stop playing.*
>
> BENJAMIN FRANKLIN

What else fills you up? What fills you up, as an adult? What do you love to do these days – that is really *just purely* for fun and joy?

What makes your soul happy? Yoga? Dancing? Long walks? Sport? Cosy nights in? Hot bubble baths? Pamper days? Time with your best friend, your partner, your kids, your dog? Cooking? Gardening? Designing?

Scribble down your thoughts and then take a real hard look at what you've got. Are you getting enough of these things in your life? Or is your life filled with things, jobs, activities and people that really *don't fill you up at all?*

If so, this could quite possibly – in fact, probably – be another underlying reason for trying to fill yourself up with food, and the root of any unwanted emotional eating habits.

I worked with a lovely Goddess called Kathryn, who is an actress living in LA. She did this exercise and found 101 amazing things that filled her up! Like spending time with her sister, going to yoga, interior design, styling and creating beautiful things, decorating and reorganizing, being outside, fashion styling, make-up…

And when we looked at her list, it was clear that acting wasn't even *on* there. The craft that she had chosen to dedicate her life to wasn't even filling her up any more. It had become a real chore for her and it turned out to be a huge factor in her unwanted eating habits. When she began to do more of the things that filled her up – got a job working as an assistant interior designer, spent more time doing yoga, stopped feeling guilty about creating things just for *fun's sake* – she took the pressure off acting – and the bingeing and emotional eating seemed to just evaporate.

Sometimes it hurts to admit that the things we have chosen to spend our lives doing just don't fill us up any more. We feel like we *should* still want it and it *should* make us happy, but the truth is – it's *totally* OK to start dabbling in other things too! So many of us have multiple passions, we shouldn't feel glued to just one.

If your life isn't filling you up – you are far more likely to turn to using food to fill you up instead.

Be the Leading Lady
in Your Own Life

You do not need anyone's permission to live the life you dream of.

You do not need to wait for someone to say 'Yep – you're now worthy. Go forth and create the life you want.'

......

That time is now, Goddess.
You can design the life you dream of.
It doesn't matter if others don't like it.
It doesn't even matter if they don't understand it.
As long as *you* like it,
As long as *you* understand it.
You, and only you, are the boss of your life.

......

If you find yourself in a story that isn't yours,
You have the right to leave.
If you find yourself in a job you hate,
A relationship that drains you,

Or a friendship that has turned toxic,
It is your right to leave.

••••••

You are in charge.
You are responsible for your happiness.
You are the leading lady in your own life.

••••••

Go spread your light into the world.
You will never feel truly 'ready'.
Nobody will come tell you when you're ready,
Ready never arrives,
Ready is now,
Go do.

Get Full of Yourself

It hurts a little, right?
If you heard someone say it about you?
'She's so full of herself!'
'She loves herself so much!'
You might say it about other women,
I've had it said about me…
And I admit, in the past I've said it about others too,
Perhaps it makes us feel better somehow.
'She's so into herself,' we say, rolling our eyes.

. . . . . .

Somewhere along the way,
You thought it would make you feel safer
To dim your light,
To fit in with the crowd,
To be liked more,
To not stand out too much,
To not live too big,
To not intimidate those around you,
To not shine too brightly,

To not be judged,
To stay where it's safe.

······

If we actually loved ourselves, or were 'full of ourselves',
What would people think?

······

I used to hate myself.
Feel broken,
Misunderstood,
Lost,
Desperate to be liked,
Desperate to fit in,
The last thing I wanted to do was love myself.
I just wanted to be liked.

······

Goddess,
You are not meant to fit in.
You are meant to fit YOU.
You are meant to be full up of yourself!
You are here to live BIG!
You are here to fall in love with yourself.
If you are not full of yourself,
If you are not in love with who you are in this world,
Who else will be?

······

You are magnificent
And it is your divine right

To be FULL of your own life,
To place your happiness in YOUR own hands,
Rather than always be looking to place it in someone else's.

· · · · · ·

You are magnificent
And it is your divine right
To fall in love with yourself.
Realize who you were born to be
And design a life you love.

· · · · · ·

You are magnificent
And it is your divine right
To say 'Yes' to yourself,
To say 'No' to the things that don't serve you,
All because you love yourself.
And know yourself
And are FULL up with your own life.

· · · · · ·

We are not here to play small, just so we don't upset or intimidate
   anyone.
We are not here to fit in, just so we don't get judged.
People will judge everything anyway – you can't help that.
The first and most important relationship of your life
Is the one with YOU.
Everything in your life
Is a mirror of that relationship.

· · · · · ·

Being full of yourself is not an insult,
It's a huge compliment.

· · · · · ·

When we are FULL of ourselves, we are full up.
We lead rich, full, abundant lives,
We are full, satisfied – happy, content, grateful.
We don't look to other things to fill us up…
(*Like food*)

· · · · · ·

So I hereby challenge you to get FULL of yourself…
Try it on for size, Goddess…

Part V

Silencing the Doubts

The only thing standing between you and your dream life and body is the BS you keep telling yourself as to why you can't do it or don't deserve it.

Meet Your Inner Skinny Bitch

She's the voice inside your head that says you need to start a diet this Monday before you get 'out of control'.

The voice that wants you to cling for dear life to a new set of rules to follow, while also telling you that you're a failure at everything you do.

The voice that calls you fat every time you walk past a shop window and the one that took over your head when you were obsessed about fitting into *that* dress for that one time. And the voice that thought it was cool to live on Diet Coke and apples all day long that time.

She's also the voice who bitches about other women. Yep – she's *that* voice! *The voice that judges other women based on their bodies.* Who compares your body to everyone else's in the room. Who tells you that you *'need'* to lose another 10lbs and made you a slave to the scales.

That voice? Why, she's your Inner Skinny B. Give her a wave. You can even give her a name if you like.

The truth is, this voice exists in every woman's head. And when we listen to her and give her power, that's when we go under.

> ### *You're not losing control – you just gave that bitch a mic and a stage.*

This bitch represents your fear of not ever being enough – good enough, skinny enough, perfect enough. This bitch is here to continually test you, and test you she shall.

Your Inner Skinny B never fully disappears – you just learn to shut her up or drown her out. Tell her where she belongs. And then she learns to pipe down and wind her neck in.

Truly, it's a skill to put her in her place every day. But the more we do it, the easier it gets.

How?

With LOVE of course!

Drown her out with thoughts and words of love, and she'll never get to win.

When she understands that you're not putting up with any more of her bullshit, she'll pipe down. She might whisper in your ear now and again, but she knows you'll just dismiss her and swipe her away like a fly flitting round your earlobe.

The moment you give her your ear, she will happily send you into a self-loathing pit of 'fat' and 'failure', and you willingly let her! You practically give yourself over to her, handcuffs and all!

Instead say, 'Bitch, you're boring me now. Change the record, seriously. I'm so over this crap you keep playing! The stuff you are coming out with is actually laughable! You really do speak so much rubbish! *La la la...* Did somebody hear something? *Boring, nobody's listening to you!* I'm seriously over this conversation already... *snoozefest.'*

Flood your thoughts full of LOVE and if you need some phrases to get you going, try any or all of these.

- I am so worthy of love!
- I feel and therefore look f*cking fabulous today!
- I am uniquely beautiful in my own way.
- I love this messy journey I am on, it's so real and gorgeous.
- Life is way too short to imprison myself.
- I love how free I feel in my body.
- I love how free I am around food, I don't spend time dwelling on it.
- I get to nourish my body with food that makes me feel and look so great.
- I am the one who gets to decide what goes in my body every day.
- I choose to talk to myself with only loving thoughts and words.

Sooner or later, your Inner Skinny B's yelling and flapping around becomes a faint whisper and a meek little voice.

My Inner Skinny B used to dominate my thoughts. Now, she goes to speak, but nothing really even comes out. She just knows I won't put up with her boring shit any more.

Your Food Story

'It takes years as a woman to unlearn what
you have been taught to be sorry for.'

AMY POEHLER

Think of all your past memories, associations and beliefs around food, weight and dieting. Think about your relationship with food as a child. Was food a reward system? Were you made to finish every last bite on your plate before you were allowed to leave the table? If so, that could be a reason for you now not listening to your body and realizing when she is full.

If you were brought up with years and years of having to finish everything on your plate, you probably have a hard time understanding when you are full or not, and you struggle to stop eating when your body is full. Again – that's totally normal! No judgement whatsoever – you are just a result of your circumstances and environment like everyone else is. But I want you to really get crystal clear. For within this story there are lessons to learn.

Think about every diet you've ever been on and how it made you feel. Every food rule you've ever set for yourself. Every meal plan you've started and everything that worked and didn't work.

Every time you ate and deep down you knew that it wasn't hunger calling you to eat.

It could be something somebody said to you about your weight? Something somebody said about your body that stuck with you – an ex-partner or boss, a work colleague, an old schoolfriend, your girlfriends – something that stuck and left an imprint on the relationship you now have with food.

It could be that subconsciously, you're using food and extra weight to feel 'protected', which may stem from an abusive or traumatic experience years ago.

Uncovering these memories can be extremely painful but all of these stories and memories make a contribution to **your story** around food and your body.

Every day you are living your life based on **your story**. It is made up of every single one of your memories, beliefs, old patterns and habits, and little things that you have learned along the way. It is what you tell yourself every day, about yourself.

For example, say you started a juice cleanse and on day two you caved and polished off an entire box of chocolates. You felt like a failure, like you were useless, like you had crap willpower – you may well be telling yourself a story of *'I don't see things through. I can't do juicing. I must be addicted to sugar.'*

And if you've failed a lot of diets in the past then you could be constantly telling yourself *'I'm a failure, I can't stick to things'*, and this could be a reason that you are constantly sabotaging your efforts to live a healthy life. Because you already believe you're incapable of seeing things through. Of course it's not *you* saying these things – it's your Inner Skinny B at work. Doing her usual tap dance.

'Named must be your fear before banish it you can.'
YODA

BS tales

Unfortunately, there's often a lot of BS in our stories. These have a massive part to play in the way you talk to yourself, the way you think about yourself and the ways in which you may be sabotaging yourself.

BS tales are, well, bullshit. The problem really arises when you start *believing* your bullshit tales to be real. For example, your story might comprise any one, or all, of the following damaging bullshit tales.

❀ I'm too big to live the life I really want.

❀ I'm never going to look like that model, so why bother?

❀ I'm useless at everything.

❀ I'm not worth cooking for, if it's just for myself.

❀ I'm not worth doing loving things for.

❀ I'm not an exercise kinda girl anyway.

❀ Life's too short to be one of those healthy people.

❀ I've got rubbish willpower.

❀ I'm crap at sticking to healthy eating.

❀ I'm not worthy of nice clothes.

❀ It's in my genes to be overweight.

❀ I've always been a sugar addict – it's who I am.

❀ I've always had problems with food, and I always will.

❀ Chocolate is my THING.

❀ I always have to order dessert, otherwise I feel like the meal isn't done.

❀

- I'm always the big one.

- If I lose weight nobody will like me.

- If I gain weight nobody will like me.

- This person is judging me because my body looks a certain way.

The challenge is to assess your story and separate the BS from the facts. So let's take a look at the above story. What is true and what is a BS tale that is holding you back from what you really want?

One of my clients did this exercise and realized that she'd been holding on to one memory years ago of being in a dance class and being called a 'big girl'. Her dance teacher had said, *'Big girls stand at the back'* – and off she had been sent to the back.

Now, what the teacher meant was 'tall' girls but, the way she heard it, she thought it meant that big girls didn't deserve to be seen, they had to stand at the back.

When she was able to see that and how meaningless it was – and actually laugh at what a load of BS it was – it freed up more space energetically for her to allow a gorgeous relationship with her body to flood back in where it deserved to be.

These BS tales are ones that you may not even realize you're using – but you keep them stored in your mind, and tell them to yourself often, without necessarily saying them out loud, which leads me to BS tales around other women.

BS tales about 'Real Women'

Now, please don't think I am saying these *are* your beliefs. I'm not at all. I'm simply throwing them out there for your dismissal, and if something stops you in your tracks then maybe you might want to ponder it for a while.

If you haven't spent your life being what you would consider a 'naturally slim woman', it's quite possible that you may have developed a few BS beliefs around how these women operate. You know, to make yourself feel better and stuff. You might not ever say these out loud or even realize they are there, or how much they could be holding you back... but here are a few BS beliefs about 'skinny women' that I've uncovered from some of the Goddesses who have opened up to me:

- ✤ 'Healthy women don't have any fun in their lives anyway.'

- ✤ 'If I was that slim I wouldn't have a social life.'

- ✤ 'I don't want to be one of those skinny women. I'm a *real* woman.'

- ✤ 'Real women have curves.'

- ✤ 'Real women are strong.'

- ✤ 'Real women know how to eat.'

- ✤ 'Real women drink beer with the guys.'

Seeing women share this kind of thing about 'real women' greatly upsets me. In case you need me to tell you, YOU, right now reading this? *You* are a real woman.

Whatever you look like. Your body shape. What you like to do in your spare time or at the gym. However much fun you have in your life. Whatever you like to drink and whoever you drink it with. Whatever your dress size. Whatever your sexuality. Got a vagina? *Congratulations.* You are officially a real woman.

But do you see how these casually thrown-around remarks could be stopping you from actually stepping into the life that you really want?

If you lost 20lbs, you'd still be a real woman. If you gained 20lbs, you'd still be a real woman.

Glad we cleared that one up. No more of this BS about who's real and who's not, please.

Deep-rooted fears

Let's not confuse BS tales with those deep-rooted fears we all have lurking somewhere. You may well have a fear that if you lose weight and become one of 'those healthy women', you might become boring or lose all of your friends. You might have a deep-rooted fear that if you *did* have the body of a healthy woman who eats well and is active, then you would also be promiscuous, flirtatious and sexually more available. And having all that extra attention could be a terrifying prospect to you. What if it meant losing your partner, or your family thinking that you think you're too good for them any more?

Do you see how these fears will constantly keep you stuck?

What are you most afraid of? What could be holding you back from living in a body you *really* love?

Only you are the author of your story. What story are you telling yourself day in day out, which is negatively affecting you and stopping you from living the life you want?

When you step into fully acknowledging your story in any given moment, you can decide to rewrite that story instantaneously.

What do you want your new story to be? How about some of the following for inspiration:

* I am worthy of having a body I love living in.

* I choose to accept myself for exactly who I am and where I am at.

- I forgive myself for carrying around these old beliefs, and now I am ready to let them go.

- I am a Goddess and I respect my body.

- I am standing in my power and it is my time.

- I deserve to be happy in my body.

- I am a healthy, happy and vibrant woman.

- I am living the life I choose.

- My body is my home for life.

- I love my body always.

- I am so much more than my reflection.

- I am so beautiful and powerful.

- I am on fire today!

- I am feeling so great!

- I love nourishing my body.

- I'm so glad I prioritize moving my body like this.

You literally can change the script in your head. What story do you want to be telling yourself every day?

Instead of telling yourself *'I don't have time to work out, I'm too busy'*, change your story to *'I'm so glad I prioritize moving my body in a way that works around my busy schedule!'*

Instead of telling yourself *'I'm a mum of two so I always have to cook for the family and put them first, which means I always end up coming last'*, change your story to *'I'm so blessed to be* a mum of two and have the opportunity to set a great example to my family by showing them how I take care of my own body'.

Of course, rewriting your story like this won't happen overnight. This is an ongoing practice. Just like infusing your day with positive thoughts and drowning out the negatives doesn't happen overnight. Talking to yourself with loving thoughts and making your story a positive one takes time, practice and lots of love. But soon enough, it will become second nature.

You are creating the world you see with your thoughts and the story you are consistently telling yourself in your head.

Goddess Corinne

'I've finally learned how to accept myself the way I am and most importantly how to love myself and to banish the self-hate.'

I could fill a whole book with my food story. It's been an emotional rollercoaster my entire life and from age six to 32 my weight went up and down like a yo-yo.

I know that I'm a sensitive soul and part of my food story is that I've never really felt loved, or learned to love myself, and have spiralled in and out of depression ever since I can remember. It has not only affected my confidence and my self-belief, but also stopped me from achieving things I so desperately want and am capable of. It's stopped me from living my life.

During the darkest times of my life, I turned to food even more and I would binge eat every day because it felt like it was the only bit of happiness and enjoyment I had. Lots of people have called me fat in the past and I've always seen myself as this fat, useless person who nobody wanted. At times, it was so bad that I turned to self-harm and even seriously considered ending my life.

Since finding Mel and the Goddesses, I've ditched all the diets. I have turned my focus away from food and on to my mind-set and self-talk to understand my emotional problems. I'm learning to be kind to myself, and making a conscious effort to love and accept myself – just the way I am. I no longer think that my weight defines me and am trying to do the best for my body, but also not beating myself up if I do eat a high-calorie meal or fancy a takeaway or some chocolate.

Best of all, I feel like I've finally let it go.

The Curse of Comparisonitis

*'From the very beginning you are being told to compare
yourself with others. This is the greatest disease; it is like
a cancer that goes on destroying your very soul because
each individual is unique, and comparison is not possible.'*

OSHO

So, how do you stop the toxic curse of comparing yourself to
every other woman in the room? Or worse – on the Internet?

Guess what? This will happen oh-so-organically when you
quit the war on You. In fact, a remarkable thing starts to happen
when we start to love ourselves. We start paying more attention
to the beauty in the other women around us, rather than judging
them and comparing traits, flaws and wobbles! We start to
worship the Goddess in others, as well as in ourselves!

'Comparison is an act of violence against the self.'

IYANLA VANZANT

A flower doesn't think of competing with the flower next to it. A rose knows it's a beautiful rose and a lily knows it's a beautiful lily. A rose will never be a lily or vice versa. But they grow alongside one another, support one another, admire one another, and allow one other to bloom fully into the most beautiful, individual flowers they can be.

Comparisonitis will hold you back beyond belief. It is a way that Your Inner Skinny B's voice can sabotage your efforts to love yourself. She will forever tell you you're not enough, you never have been and you never will be. She also loves to compare you with every other girl on the Internet or in the room, based on how pretty, thin, successful or smart she may be.

This voice doesn't simply vanish overnight. I have done a lot of work on loving myself, loving my body and shutting that little voice out – but she still finds a way to shimmy on through the cracks sometimes. She's a sneaky bugger.

It has taken time, but I now genuinely love living in my body and that's with practice and commitment always to let the love in. Negative thoughts creep in from time to time – about myself, my abilities or my body – but I constantly shut them down completely by telling them they are unwelcome. I never let them transcend into anything significant. Instead I challenge them to come forth and manifest if they would be so brave, but they never do because the voice of love (your soul, your truth) outweighs the fear (your ego, your doubts).

If you find yourself comparing your abilities, your work or your body to another woman, first observe and acknowledge what's happening. Then calmly ask yourself, 'What am I feeling, why has this been brought up and where has it come from?'

What in this other woman has triggered you? What parts of you are feeling vulnerable or threatened by her presence that you can make sense of? This is not about the woman. She is just being herself. *It is about you.* It's highly likely that the parts that you feel triggered by, the parts that are making you compare yourself, are parts that you already have inside of you.

Recognize that the other woman is you. The parts in her that trigger you are parts within you that you also have. Maybe they are parts you abandoned, or maybe they are parts you have suppressed.

As always, when you can get really honest about how you feel – without holding back – it usually clears up a lot of unanswered questions, and you're able to become your own detective.

Then allow the love to flood back in.

Nobody can compare to her. She is so beautiful and charming. Her very soul just lights up the room. It's not her make-up. Nor the clothes she wears. Not her hair. Not her bum. Not the photos she posts. But how she is unapologetically herself. That is what's irreplaceable. And it makes her shine so bright. Nobody can compare, because nobody is her. Other women are no threat to her. There is only one of her in the world. And that's what makes her so beautiful. And that's what makes YOU beautiful, too.

You are her and she is you.

When you are unapologetically authentic, there is no comparison.

We are all beautiful and we are all the same.

*You are not in competition
with anyone.*

*Another woman's beauty doesn't
make you less beautiful.*

*Another woman's intelligence
doesn't make you less smart.*

*Another woman's success
doesn't make you a failure.*

*Stop competing with the
Goddesses around you.*

*We are all unique and
we are all beautiful.*

*There is no competition when
you are being yourself!*

Celebrity Culture

Look at any of the women's gossip magazines and you're likely to find the following 'stories'.

Front page: **Find out what celebrities really weigh!**

Page 4: **Stars flaunt their 'new curves' on the beach!**

Page 6: **The latest celebrity fad diet!**

Page 12: **New study says chocolate and wine can aid weight loss!**

Page 20: **How to lose 4kg in seven days for your beach holiday!**

Page 24: **What's in this celebrity's fridge?**

Page 30: **Fear for star who looks 'too skinny', friends worry she has 'gone too far'!**

Back pages: **Plastic surgery ads.**

It's just another way we love to compare ourselves to other women. Women in the media. Women in magazines. Women we watch on TV, stalk on the Internet, ogle at on billboards.

Let's take gossip magazines as one example – how do you feel flicking through these magazines and being forced to compare yourself to these women? Truthfully?

These recognized Goddesses – who we have put in the public eye – are real people, you know. Can you actually even begin to imagine having your body splashed all over the front page of these magazines and then scrutinized and picked apart and ogled by hundreds of thousands of women every day? (After all, let's be honest, men don't buy these magazines to read. It's us.)

Can you actually imagine there being a male equivalent of these magazines and tabloids? Men critiquing other men's bodies and talking about who has a six-pack and who has a beer gut? Who's gained 5kg this winter and who lost it? Photos of them in their Speedos, 'flaunting their bodies' on the beach? (*How very dare they!*)

No. Of course you can't imagine it because it's utterly ridiculous, that's why. And yet for us women this behaviour has become completely the norm.

> *Avoid filling your head with trash and you'll be less likely to fill your body with trash. The two go hand in hand.*

If you want to be your happiest, most vibrant and healthy self, really think about what you are fuelling your *mind* with as well as your body. What are you reading and seeing? Are you filling your head with positive, encouraging thoughts? Are you teaching yourself something worthwhile? Are you helping yourself move forwards or backwards, or staying stuck in comparisonitis?

Stop buying magazines that encourage body negativity and constant judgement. What do you actually expect to happen inside *your* head when you look through them? How do you think this will affect your food choices, and the relationship you have with your body?

What thoughts do you want to be filling your mind with?

It is actually a dream of mine to have a regular column in a women's magazine and be a positive influence on the women reading it – and help to transform the way they view themselves and their bodies. Weekly self-love, body love, lifting women up instead of tearing them down! Positive affirmations, some great recipes, of course, and an advice and Q&A section. After all the damage that has been done, this is so needed!

Isn't it about time we started praising the women we have put in the spotlight rather than tearing them down and searching for flaws?

Isn't it about time we supported each other as sisters and fellow Goddesses?

Isn't it about time we realized that the beauty of another woman doesn't subtract from *our own* beauty?

Love and praise the women in the spotlight and public eye, just as you should love and praise the Goddesses around you.

And read fewer gossip magazines, more books!

Insta-perfect
Highlight Reel Lives

It's no secret that we are living in the era of Instagram, Facebook, Snapchat and everything filtered, edited and showcased online in the best possible light and at the best possible angle.

I recently heard about a yoga blogger, Photoshopping their pictures to make their bodies look thinner or more 'perfect'. In the same week, I also heard about how a famous food blogger spends hours getting the perfect shot of their crazy-amazing rainbow smoothie – with the perfect drizzles coming down the side of a perfect mason jar – and then throwing it out because, behind the lens, she is battling with a crippling eating disorder and this is her way of 'dealing with it'.

Both on the surface appear to be a leading a super-healthy and vibrant lifestyle, drinking healthy smoothies, doing yoga poses and cooking up big delicious dishes.

Both of these stories were deeply upsetting to me and really struck a chord, and made me start questioning a lot about the way we act online. *How much of what we see on social media is actually real at all?*

When I first started blogging about food in 2012, I was sharing pictures of beautiful green smoothies and vegan meals. I didn't share how I was still obsessively weighing myself, still hated my body and often binged on processed vegan junk food, instead of eating real food or having proper meals.

We know by now that Instagram and Facebook posts are simply the highlight reels of everyone's lives, and never the full story.

You might share a photo of you looking great at a party. But would you post one of you at the end of the night when you were completely plastered, and needed to be put in a taxi home?

You would maybe share a photo of you and your boyfriend looking super-happy and relaxed together, but would you post one of when you're going through really hard times and constantly fighting with each other?

You perhaps can't wait to share a photo of your body when you've been really hitting the gym and just completed a detox. But would you post one when you've just eaten 'til you thought you were about to pop?

The food blogger probably doesn't share the junk food she eats on the weekend, only the healthy meals she prepares and makes photo-ready Monday to Friday.

The model who posts three selfies a day with perfect, glowing skin may actually be struggling with acne all over her face, but edits her selfies with an app, so she has the perfect complexion in photos.

The travel blogger may show herself on a beach in a bikini having a blast, but doesn't show that she's in a hotel room at night crippled with loneliness because she has nobody to share her experiences with apart from her 100K followers and the photographer she hired.

The fashion blogger may show herself kitted out in expensive designer clothes and handbags for her 'OOTD' – but wouldn't share that she is actually in thousands of dollars' worth of credit-card debt and has no idea how she is going to pay her rent this month.

Models might show photos of themselves having a blast on yachts in the South of France, but they certainly don't show the photo of the old rich guy who actually owns the yacht!

Obviously I'm generalizing and using stereotypes here – but you get my point.

I often receive messages on Facebook from people who say things like, *'Wow Mel, everything looks like it's amazing for you! You're living the dream!'*

While I am grateful to live a life I truly adore 99.9 per cent of the time... and most of my posts generally try to reflect this by being positive, uplifting and happy – I am still a real person, who also goes through shit times. Sometimes I read these messages and feel guilty for posting stuff that could be perceived to be 'perfect' in somebody else's eyes because, behind the scenes, my life is *far* from perfect, just like yours.

I feel very strongly that women who have a following on social media have a certain amount of *responsibility* to let their followers see their real lives, not just their fake 'shiny' ones from their highlight reel.

Like most bloggers, my reasons for not posting the *'part I didn't post'* up until now is that I want my posts to be **positive, uplifting and empowering** to those who see them. And I'm also a big believer in that energetically you get more of what you give out! So in order to attract more of the good stuff into my life, I share what I am grateful for and what makes me happy – not what I am upset or aggravated over.

However, outing my struggles with food and eating disorders not only helped me gain closure but also helped thousands of other Goddesses. So it was worth it a million per cent! Here are some examples of my own highlight reel posts versus my actual reality.

Highlight reel: I had a blast on a six-week solo adventure in New York, California and Miami! I'm having the time of my life!

I didn't post: Earlier in the year I had been through the devastating breakdown of my marriage. I booked that six-week trip when I decided I was done with crying every day. The truth is I felt like my life had fallen apart. That solo trip was an act of self-love to help me discover my true self, and what I wanted from this new chapter of my life.

Highlight reel: I had an amazing time in Joshua Tree, California, stayed in a gorgeous log cabin and hiked up a mountain! (And took loads of cool photos from the top of the mountain!)

I didn't post: The night before I took that awesome photo of me doing yoga on a mountain, I woke up in tears in the middle of the night because I had a vivid dream about a conversation I was having with my late dad. For those of you who have lost a parent, sibling or someone close to you, you will know – those nights don't go away.

Highlight reel: I love being an adventurer! I love travelling! I'm such a free spirit!

I didn't post: I also still sometimes get bouts of anxiety when I'm away from home, and often can feel unsettled and struggle to ground myself. Travelling can be a real test of strength for me and has taught me how I can easily stop looking after myself when I'm away from the comforts of my home.

Highlight reel: I have a lot of moments of 'I love my life so much!' and I practice gratitude every single day.

I didn't post: Sometimes I still have days where I'm so overwhelmed I just want to curl up and hide under the covers all day and not show up in my life at all. Yep! I have those days too.

Highlight reel: I have a lot of friends all around the world. I'm a social butterfly!

I didn't post: Sometimes I really just don't want to be around anyone whatsoever. I want to go into my own little bubble and just reflect by myself and recharge my batteries alone and not have any human contact. And I think it's absolutely OK to do that.

Highlight reel: Photos of healthy food in New York.

I didn't post: Photos of all the cocktails I drank there too, and the calamari and tacos I ordered a few times late at night. I didn't post about that, because it's not beautiful or healthy, and wouldn't inspire anyone else to lead healthier and happier lives. But – it sure as hell happened!

I also reached out to some of my blogger friends to ask them to do the same and share some highlight reels versus the reality! Here are some of the super-interesting responses I got...

'I used to blog about fashion, beauty, and generally living as glamorously as my graduate income would allow. But I didn't write about how my boyfriend was verbally, emotionally and ultimately physically abusing me.'

GABRIELLA, FASHION BLOGGER

'I'd be lying if I said I didn't feel under pressure to present myself and my lifestyle in a certain way. I forget looking at other people's blogs and social media profiles that they probably worry about it too. Everything goes through a filter! And I'll primp, reposition, and tweak things from my hair parting to the words on the post. It's never as effortless as it looks.'

LUCY, LIFESTYLE BLOGGER

'My blog is all based on being a healthy mom. And, yes, I do those things but the reality is for every nice moment we have, there's always lots of tears and tantrums and stress! People always say they don't know how I do it because I make everything from scratch, but I have to because of my son's allergies – and although the food looks pretty in the photo, my kitchen is a complete tip! I also still have the battle of my kids wanting junk food. On Instagram I post pictures of them eating healthy food but I don't post a picture of the battle I've had in the grocery store trying to get candy off him!'

TANYA, FOOD BLOGGER

'For every yoga picture that makes it onto my Instagram feed I have 200 fails!'

SASHA, YOGA BLOGGER

'It's often the most perfect-looking people and relationships that are plastered all over social media that have the most insecurities or hidden problems behind the scenes. I for one have always been a happy, smiley,

*confident character who always posts positive photos, but
as a result of this behaviour and confidence, no one tends
to ask me if I am OK, or ask how things are going on in my
life, as they think it is so perfect from the images I post.'*

HANNAH, FOOD BLOGGER

*'Instagram sees a fraction of my life. It doesn't see
my Batman PJs that my mum picked up for me from
Asda, or the fact I spilled tomato juice all down my
top today whilst watching an old rerun of Friends. It
doesn't see my meltdowns. It doesn't see that the
perfect marble flat lay is actually a cheap roll of sticky-
back plastic shoved to the side of my dresser.'*

ZOE, BEAUTY BLOGGER

You heard it from them, guys. Don't take social media seriously.
Spend less time glued to your phone. Hide the apps. Catch
yourself scrolling and make yourself do something else that will
make you feel great about yourself.

*Real life is what happens behind
the lens, not in front of it.*

*When the phone stays in the bag
because you're having such a good
time you forget to take photos.*

Live free from comparisonitis – and live a gorgeously messy,
unretouched life behind the lens.

#Fitspiration

'I have insecurities, of course, but I don't hang out with anyone who points them out to me.'

ADELE

If you follow these kind of social media fitness accounts (and there are thousands) then it's kinda like hanging out with these people, every day, or every time you look at your phone.

Ask yourself, 'Are they *really* motivating you? Are they making you feel *good* about your life? Or are they actually making you feel worse, like a failure, inadequate, like you're not enough. Like you need to have washboard abs and a big round butt in order to be *enough*?'

If there were people in your *real* life that were constantly making you feel bad about yourself, inadequate, like a failure, then would you keep them in your life? Hopefully not. Hopefully you'd ditch them.

Treat your online world the same.

Unfollow the people who don't build you up, but make you chase perfection instead. Inspiration is a beautiful thing, but actually ask yourself *honestly* if these accounts have helped you move forwards so far in your journey when it comes to health and fitness? Have they helped? Or have they only made you hate your own body more?

It's perfectly OK to want to change your body, but in order to get the body you want, you have to start by loving and respecting the body you have.

You can't hate yourself happy, and comparing your body to someone else's doesn't make it change.

The Price of Perfection

*'Perfectionism is a twenty-ton shield that
we lug around thinking it will protect us
when, in fact, it's the thing that's really
preventing us from taking flight.'*

BRENÉ BROWN

Perfectionism is destroying your spirit.
Slowly.

......

I know it feels great when the scales are on your side.
When you're making meticulously controlled, perfect choices, all
    in line with your plan.
You feel so powerful that day.
So in control.
So virtuous.
But when you eat something not perfect,
Or heaven forbid, gain a pound or two,
Your whole world crumbles and you fall apart.
I know it's not fun to live on that rollercoaster.

I know how great you feel when you've been riding all the way to
  the top
But as soon as you're there
You know you're coming down –
Fast...
And it's horrible to see you go through it, day after day,
Week after week,
Year after year.

......

But please don't panic.
We actually all *know* you're not perfect.
But here's a secret. None of us are.
No – not even those girls that you think are.
It's actually quite *impossible* to be perfect,
And perfect isn't a number.
I know you think when you reach your goal,
Then you'll be happy
But Goddess you won't...
I guarantee you won't.
What will bring you happiness is not a number.
What will bring you happiness is total and complete freedom.

......

Freedom from the quest of perfection.
Freedom from this battle you keep fighting.
Because perfectionism is a full-time job!
But you're not getting paid – you're just a full-time volunteer.
And you put so much time and effort into it.
It takes up all your headspace,
And you have a whole life that is waiting for you...

Waiting for you to go out and live it,
And make mistakes,
And have fun,
And make a mess,
And make things up as you go along sometimes.

......

We love when you do that.
We love when you laugh.
We love when you go with the flow.
We love when you surrender and just wing it sometimes.
We love when you allow yourself to enjoy life!
It's so beautiful.
We fall in love with you when you are unapologetically being
    yourself.
When you are enjoying life to the max.

......

Nobody cares if you have a perfect intake.
Nobody cares if you hit your goal weight.
Did you know, when you're busy trying to be perfect,
Your friends and family wonder where you have disappeared off
    to?
While you're off in your own world, counting, tracking, worrying,
Beating yourself up…

......

All we want is for you to be free.
It's time to come home.
It's time to let your light shine bright again.
Fabulous, flawed, imperfect.
Beautifully, unapologetically you.

••••••

We know you're not perfect, Goddess.
It's OK – neither are we.

••••••

Your best is good enough.
Stop the fight.
Surrender to the beauty and the chaos that is life.

••••••

…And now that you don't need to be perfect,
You can be real.

One of the most powerful forms of self-love is to give yourself a million second chances when you mess up. Everyone messes up, all the time. The beauty is being able to forgive yourself straight away, and swiftly get over it so you can move on with your life.

Be Gentle with Yourself, You're Doing Your Best

It's true, we don't have a full understanding of what actually goes into our food. That's an understatement. We read articles about what goes into our foods in terms of chemicals, pesticides, preservatives – but what can we do about it without becoming obsessed with every morsel we put into our mouths?

Eat locally grown, fresh and organic produce where you can, cook meals from scratch as much as you can, and make choices that your body will feel nourished by.

But you can't eat 100 per cent perfect.

It's OK if you don't live 100 per cent organic.

It's OK if you don't live a life with zero processed foods in whatsoever.

It's OK if you buy vegetables that aren't organic, or eat salted nuts instead of raw, or eat pasta or bread or even a creamy sauce one time, despite you knowing it's not the most nutritionally beneficial food in the world.

In fact, it's not physically possible to follow every single rule about food you ever read on the Internet. It's simply not doable. Yes, check the ingredients on your food, but don't get obsessed with it. If you live your entire life this way, sooner or later you will have completely sucked the joy out of eating – and it becomes a real struggle and 'chore' for you to do – rather than a happy, fun experience.

Being healthy is not just about the food, but having a healthy mind-set around the food. For that, you absolutely 100 per cent *have to accept the fact* that there is no such thing as a perfect diet – and you won't be able to eat 100 per cent perfectly all of the time.

The trick to being happy and healthy with your food is to let balance, flexibility and acceptance be your guiding principles. And remember – your best is good enough.

Goddess Helen

'What I've found is that the kinder I am towards myself and my body, the more self-assured I feel and the less I am afraid to show my body off and just be me.'

I feel like I didn't find Mel – she found me when she popped up in my Facebook feed. Until then, dieting ruled my life. Simple, I was either on a strict diet and feeling OK or off the diet and binge eating. Neither made me feel good about myself nor happy.

I hated the way my body looked and that ended up marring what should have been a beautiful day – our wedding. We had beautiful photographs but I couldn't face looking at the album – it was too hard to look at pictures of me without pulling them apart and criticizing them. It put an enormous strain on our relationship and, after giving birth to our son, things got worse.

Needless to say my postpartum body didn't match up to the ones in the magazines and suddenly I longed to have the body back – the one I'd previously hated. I almost resented our son for damaging my body and was too body conscious to reveal her to my husband, let alone anyone else.

Our son is now two years old and in the last six months I've experienced a massive transformation. I no longer see food as 'bad' and 'good' and am now eating so much more healthily – I've even replaced my Diet Coke addiction with green juices!

I've started to feel more confident about myself and my body. I'm no longer afraid to look at photos of myself and even went on a spa day with my husband to celebrate our second wedding anniversary – I would never have done that before! I still don't like my stretch marks but I've learned to accept them… they're part of me and tell the story of my son's birth – and I just love that.

. . . .

You may be so used to
dissecting your features,
that you have no idea
how beautiful you
look to a stranger.

How to Stop Scrutinizing Photos

Are you someone who dissects every photo of yourself that you see, scrutinizing and criticizing your body, and so consistently reinforcing feelings of being 'not good enough'?

I used to agonize over every photo of myself, and seeing a bad photo would cause such stress, anxiety and self-loathing. I would even go as far to say that a bad photo of myself would completely ruin my night. How very sad.

And let us not forget the female posing rules…

* Is this my best side?

* Does my arm look skinny at this angle?

* Are my legs positioned right?

* Is my belly sucked in?

* Should I stick my bum out more?

Can you imagine if when your friend got out the phone to take a photo on a night out, you and your girlfriends actually just *carried* on having a great time, stood together and smiled like you meant it? Rather than popping your hip, positioning your legs, sticking an arm on your hip, before demanding that more photos be taken 'til you're all happy?

It seriously disturbs me how I can look back at old photos and immediately know exactly what I weighed at that time, what particular method or diet I had been using in an attempt to try to manipulate my body, what rules I was following, and mainly *how I felt about myself* when that photo was taken.

I don't remember the great times I had, the things people said to me that night, the hysterical belly laughs or the fun, exciting memories. I mean, I do – but those memories are all overshadowed by *how I felt about myself*. I should have been having the time of my life and loving every second of it – the parties, the photos, the events. But instead, I was consumed with self-loathing and feelings of discomfort in my own body.

What a sad waste. I will never get that time back.

If you can relate to this, then I'm sure you too can look back at photos from a big family event, whether it's Christmas Day or a friend's party, and remember how you felt in your body.

Does it tarnish the happy memory that the photo was supposed to be capturing?

Do you look at photos of happy memories and cringe at how you look, instead of reliving that day and feeling joy?

If you relate to this, then you might find the following four steps helpful.

1. Look at you as a *whole* person. You are so used to picking yourself and your features apart, you have no idea how beautiful you are as a whole person.

2. Remember *you are not your body*. When did we become a nation of women who judged and critiqued ourselves purely

on appearance? Think about the people you love most in your life. I'm sure they are absolutely gorgeous to you. Is it about their looks though? Do you care what shape their body is, or if they have a crooked smile in a photo or if they have a belly bulge? I'll bet it doesn't even cross your mind for a second. *You are so much more than just your body.* You are a unique, beautiful human, with so much to give in this lifetime. So much more than just the way your outer shell appears in one photo.

3. Take fewer photos of yourself. *Be more present instead.* I used to take a gazillion photos every time I went on a night out, but I have actually noticed recently that I have a *much* better night if I'm not constantly taking photos. I try now to capture more feelings and experiences in the photos I do take.

4. Be present with your friends. *Relish the entire experience.* Did you have an amazing night with your best girlfriends? Did you dance 'til 3 a.m.? Did someone say or do something that night that had you in fits of hysterical laughter? Did you experience something incredible? Did you have a really special, heart-warming moment with a family member? Did you catch up with someone you love whom you haven't seen in forever?

> **Don't look back at photos next month or next year having completely forgotten the evening apart from how you were sucking in your belly all night.**

You might also want to…

❖ Make a commitment to go to events and *just* have fun.

❖ Focus on the memory-making moments and don't let yourself get caught up in how you think you look, or how you can hide from the camera.

❖ Go back and look at your photos and find ones that make you cringe a little, or you'd normally skip over because you think your belly looks too big, and rewrite that story. Think about how much *fun* you had, how great it was to see your friends or to be there making new ones!

Rewrite the memory in a brand new, positive light.

Don't lose out on those memories because you're consumed with thoughts around your food or your weight. Those beautiful, real experiences only come around once.

Thin Does Not Equal Happy

It's a common belief that the thinner you get, the more you should like yourself. But the truth is:

* 'Thin' women can look in the mirror and hate what they see, or they can love it.

* 'Fat' women can look in the mirror and hate what they see, or they can love it.

* 'Normal' women can look in the mirror and hate what they see, or they can love it.

* 'Real' women can look in the mirror and hate what they see, or they can love it.

We have been told for years after years, whole lifetimes for some of us, that being thin equals happiness. This is something we're sold with every TV advert for a diet plan, the promised celeb diet secrets on the covers of magazines and even the choice of women for clothing advertising and runway models. We're constantly being told that this is what we should want. All of it has added up to this blanket belief that we are only successful if we are thin, and that being thin should make us happy.

It's all too easy to think that the grass is greener on the other side of the diet, but if you're not happy with yourself now, you won't be happy with yourself there. Wherever you go, there you are. That is why we must work on our relationship with food and our body, rather than just continue trying desperately to change our body with diets, and expecting lifelong happiness and contentment to appear suddenly.

Goddess Sally

'Looking back, I would have never thought this achievable, but I'm here!'

I started to gain weight when I was 15 and by the time I was 17 weighed 11st 7lbs – which seemed a lot on my 5ft 3in frame. I just wanted to be like all the other teens I knew – to go out and have fun with my friends – so turned to the latest fad diet for help. I just wanted my clothes to fit, to feel good about myself, I didn't intend to punish myself or be labelled 'anorexic' but that – in the end – is what happened.

I went on an extreme carb-free diet and before I knew it was down at my 'ideal' weight. Fantastic, right? No, because I still wasn't happy and so pushed on and on with the diet. Each year eating less and losing more. By the time I was 24, I'd pretty much given up eating altogether and weighed a fraction of my former weight. I was also in hospital several times a week with horrendous panic attacks, my clothes were children's sizes, my face was long and crusty and my hip bones rubbed sore on any trousers I wore. I knew my parents were terrified for me but I just didn't know how to stop. I didn't know how get back to just eating normally again.

Then one day, in the car on the way to the hospital (again), I heard my dad say 'Oh Sal… what's happening to my family?' And something burst inside of me. I'd forgotten that I was not only affecting myself, but also the people who MADE me. Who loved me! Those words changed everything and I decided to seek help – and start listening. I cried a river in the doctor's consultation room but being diagnosed with an eating disorder and told to 'talk about my problems' wasn't the fix I needed. I had a happy home life and didn't have problems. I'd just forgotten how to eat normally. I'd stopped listening to my body and I didn't know how to get back on the road to health.

Then I found Mel. She knew exactly what I needed: re-educating to love my body and fuel it with the right foods. She understood that I wasn't broken! I didn't need fixing!

Everything has changed since that day. Food is now nourishment, enjoyment and love, as opposed to an inconvenience and scary. It has a major purpose and is ultimately interesting. I know how to use it, and I know how to appreciate it. The exact same words apply to my body too. For what it is, with its blips and quirks, it's me and MINE. I'm cherishing it now. My parents gave me this gift and I'm not going to waste it.

. . . .

How do you expect to
love yourself, if you're
not being yourself?

Are You Being YOU?

'Can you remember who you were, before
the world told you who you should be?'
Danielle LaPorte

It's fairly impossible to love yourself if you're not *being* yourself.

With every chapter of your life, you should be learning and discovering new things about *you* and who you are, what makes you tick and what serves you to be living at your highest potential.

Perhaps you only did that degree because it would get you a 'good job'. Perhaps you choose not to wear red lipstick and bright pink heels in case people think you're 'too much'. Perhaps you really want bright red hair but are worried what people would think of you.

Do you feel like you're able to be absolutely, unapologetically, *you* right now? Do you feel like you are surrounded by people who are supporting you and encouraging you to be the best version of yourself – *all* of you? The highs, the lows, and everything in between?

If you came out with all the things that truly light you up and started living the life you dreamed of, would you support yourself and *really* believe in yourself? I mean – fully and completely? Would the people you choose to spend time with support *all* of you, if you let your real self be seen? Or do you feel like you're suppressing a part of yourself that is absolutely desperate to get out and show itself?

If you feel like you're still trying to fit in, trying to be liked, and not fully expressing who you are, then this could well be a potential cause of unwanted food habits. Using food as a way to suppress the feeling of being…well, suppressed.

Have you ever felt like you were suppressing who you truly are deep down, or living in a story that isn't meant to be yours? Or like you're playing a certain 'role' rather than just being *fully, completely and beautifully YOU?*

I've felt like this several times in my life. I've felt like I had to fit a certain role, stereotype, look, persona.

On the surface, I was quite happy and content with these different roles. I went out of my way to be happy. I threw myself into it, well and truly. Threw everything at it. But the niggle was there. The feeling of suppressing who I really was.

Run towards anything or anyone who makes you feel like you are coming home to YOURSELF.

What parts of your life are not bringing out the best in you? What can you let fall away? If you are spending time with people who are not bringing out good qualities in you, it's OK to start distancing yourself. It's an act of self-love.

Dabble, create, inspire and be inspired. Before you know it, you'll be attracting the life of your dreams into your reality, and using food as a weapon to beat yourself with will no longer be an option. It may not even be a conscious shift at first, but it could be the most rewarding thing you will ever do for your body.

Get ready to start living the life of your dreams, because suddenly, you will feel empowered, intuitive, invincible. You will have completely stepped into your truth.

'In the world through which you travel,
you are endlessly creating yourself.'
FRANTZ FANON

People Pleasing

When you begin to say NO to the things you don't want to do, or the people you don't want to be around, you begin to say **YES to yourself** and living your truth.

I actually think 'no' is an extremely underused word, and we should use it more often.

That's not to say you should be letting your friends down, being flaky or unreliable. It's just to say that you need to truly ask yourself more often, 'Is this what I really want to do, *or* am I trying to make others happy here, neglecting what I truly want?'

I know that there are times where we have to do things that we don't particularly find exciting or interesting, and that's one thing. But you can seriously minimize how often that is by respecting yourself enough to say no, when people expect too much from you and push your boundaries, or you know you will resent it later on, even if you keep it bottled up.

Often we go along with things that we really don't want to do because we are so damn scared of upsetting anyone. And that can be a *huge* trigger for emotional eating for *many* women, because they suppress their own needs and just continue to give, give, give.

You can't give from an empty cup.

If you're a mum who feels like you have no time to yourself because you're constantly running around after your kids, then have a look at what you can delegate and where you can start saying no on some occasions. Can you hire a cleaner? Share lifts with another parent? Can you drop your kids at their grandma's house one night a week, so you and your partner can go on a date and enjoy each other? Bring your Future You life into your reality.

One of the biggest reasons why we overeat, or emotionally eat, can be feeling like we are trying to be someone we are not. So if you're *doing* something that you really don't *want* to do – e.g. being in a job you don't like, a relationship you don't want to be in, constantly giving in a friendship and never receiving – that can be a huge trigger to turn to food. And when you start looking at how you spend your time – and how a vast amount of time might be spent doing things you really resent doing – that could be a huge catalyst for ending your unwanted eating patterns for good, too.

You are worth it.

When have you been saying YES when you should have been saying NO? What can you delegate to someone else or let fall away? And what have you done lately just to please *you* and you only?

When we're in a constant state of pleasing others, giving out our energy to things that don't fill us up, we can become so drained of energy that we accrue an energetic debt. *Nobody can pay off that debt for us. We have to find a way to pay it back to ourselves.*

And just like paying off a financial debt, it is best done little and often – rather than letting the debt get so bad that you wind up in a complete mess and unable to keep your head above water.

Go to your diary and start brainstorming things in your life right now that you can actually say no to. Free up more room in your life for stuff that you *really do* want in your ideal life. Then recharge your batteries by yourself, little and often, by doing what fills you up and gives you joy. Things that make you feel good about being you. I honestly can't tell you how much doing this can impact on your relationship with food and your body. Why? Because it is a constant message to your body that says, *'You are worth it!'*

**By saying NO more to the things
that don't fill you up, you say YES
to you, and the things that do.**

Goodbye FOMO – Embrace Your JOMO

'Nobody really cares if you don't go to the party.'
Courtney Barnett

JOMO, meaning 'Joy of Missing Out', is the opposite of the commonly used acronym FOMO, 'Fear of Missing Out'.

If you're someone who says yes to every invitation, attends every party, every social occasion, every event, because you can't bear the thought of missing out or not being involved, then it may be that you're plagued with FOMO. But, guess what? You don't actually *have* to go at all. You don't even have to come up with an amazing excuse. You can actually choose to stay at home and paint your nails instead and get an early night. Life hack:

You literally do not have to do all the things or be at all the places.

Isn't that a relief?

Living constantly on the go, we risk serious burnout and stress, so being mindful of the life we are creating has never been more important.

There will always be more parties, more networking events, more dinners. These will never go away. The people you so badly *need* to catch up with will still be there next week.

There will *never* be a day when you sit down and say, or think, 'You know, I'm all caught up with everyone I needed to catch up with! I can now relax.' That day will never come.

This not about being a flaky friend or letting people down, it's about not letting *yourself* down by saying yes to everything only because of your FOMO. It's about being clear on how you want to feel. And sometimes that means saying no to the party in favour of staying in, getting an early night and reflecting on your life, your thoughts and where you want to be heading.

The truth is, your true friends will understand when you need time alone to recharge your batteries and will appreciate you putting that first.

I always encourage my Goddesses to take themselves on regular self-dates. Show up somewhere alone or book into a workshop or event. Heaven forbid – go out for dinner or to see a movie alone! Don't be embarrassed about it – be empowered by it, and develop a newfound appreciation for your own company.

If you can truly let go of your need to be 'involved' all the time, it's so good for your soul to take a break from other people and just be connected with yourself and your thoughts. This is your time for you. To reflect on anything that might have come up lately in your personal life, rather than go out and distract yourself from it.

Time alone is time spent getting to know you.

*It's your time to chill out, catch up on rest,
and spend time nurturing yourself.*

When my eating habits were at their worst, I also noticed I was terrified of being alone. Overeating seemed to distract me from my loneliness, my anxiety and my fear of being unloved. I would drag any friend I could along to dinner that night, or to the movies, or anywhere in fact – just so I didn't have to be home alone with my destructive thought patterns.

What I didn't realize was that in neglecting time by myself I was making the problem 100 times worse, and facing the thing I feared – being alone – might have got me on the path to healing quicker. But instead, I was in self-destruct mode and my weapon of choice was food. Food and alcohol, in fact. I was at every party, every event, every dinner, every 'let's do drinks'.

Putting your JOMO into action is easier than you think, too. Take last Halloween, for example, when I let my FOMO slide – and accepted the fact that I needed a weekend to myself instead of wriggling into a mermaid costume and meeting up with friends. Despite really not wanting to miss out on all the fun, I just knew that I needed time to catch up with myself and rest. My friends were great about it and luckily mermaids don't go out of style, so I was happy to put my costume away for next year.

Here's what I did instead:

* Went to two yoga classes.

* Wrote 10,000 words of this book.

* Decluttered, cleaned out and organized my kitchen cupboards.

* Caught up with sleep, emails, laundry and admin.

- Made my home feel beautiful by cleaning it top to bottom, then lit incense sticks and candles.

- Made a huge batch of carrot and coconut soup.

It truly does give you a strong sense of contentment to be able to say no rather than always be the person saying yes.

If you said yes to everyone who wanted to meet you for a coffee, dinner, lunch, brunch, you would have zero time left for *you* that week. Zero time left for yourself, to recharge your batteries.

So I invite you to place your FOMO aside, and instead, embrace your JOMO. Create a calm space for reflection and actually prioritizing what is important to you right now.

You won't lose friends, you won't miss out; there will always be more invitations. What's more, when you embrace your JOMO, you value your time and decide exactly where your energy should be spent, which means other people will value it too.

Confidence is not
'They will like me.'

Confidence is 'I'll be
OK if they don't.'

Fear of Being Judged by Others

*'Do what you feel in your heart to be right
– for you'll be criticized anyway.'*

ELEANOR ROOSEVELT

It is a sad truth that we spend a lot of time seriously concerned about what other people think of us and our actions. Our fear of being judged by others plays a huge part in why we don't do the things in our life we really want to do, or go after our dream lives!

Something I wish I'd known growing up, is that people will judge you regardless of what you do, so you may as well do what *you* want to do, whether they like it or not, or whether they even understand it or not. You can't escape judgement. Nobody goes through life never getting judged by anyone.

*'To avoid criticism – do nothing,
say nothing, be nothing.'*

ELBERT HUBBARD

The truth is, most people are generally so wrapped up in their own lives that they *genuinely don't care that much* what others are doing with theirs. People may see you do your thing, pass judgement for a brief, fleeting moment but then – essentially – they will *carry on living their own lives*. No one is judging you anywhere *near* as much as you are actually judging yourself.

If you think about it, it's also really none of your business what other people think of you at all. What truly matters is how you think of *yourself*. So get over your fear of being judged – by loving yourself without judgement.

When you stop judging yourself, you rise above any judgement from others.

Other People and Their Stuff

'It is impossible to live a life of authenticity without pissing a few people off along the way.'

BRENÉ BROWN

When you start to get conscious around your eating habits and food patterns, and start to live a healthier life, you will undoubtedly notice other people throwing their stuff at you. By throwing their stuff, I mean projecting their relationship with food or their body onto you.

When other women are judgemental of your choices around food, your body, your weight – it is simply them speaking from *their* experiences, *their* environment, *their* relationship with food. *Their* story and limiting beliefs. *Their stuff*.

We are all just a result of our experiences, our conditioning and our environment.

Often when groups of women get together and talk food, weight, diets, body image, etc. – all that comes together is a huge accumulation of *everyone's* stuff. And that's a *lot of stuff to deal with*.

It's no wonder we wind up feeling overwhelmed. As soon as we start a new diet, we then have to hear what Sally, Laura, Mary and Sue all think about nutrition, what diets **they're** trying, or what so-and-so is eating lately.

But remember this, my friend, nobody – *nobody* – is the expert of your body except YOU.

So when you speak with a friend about your food, your diet, your body, your weight – you are quite often choosing to accept to take on *all their stuff too*. It's no surprise that doing this can leave us way more overwhelmed than we were to start off with.

So focus on your own stuff. Don't let other women give you their stuff to carry around too.

If they do – simply send it back. Visualize yourself saying to this person, *'Thanks so much for offering me all your stuff, but I'm gonna send it straight back to you and focus on my own instead.'*

We are all creatures of love. And anything that is not said with love is actually often just a call for love.

When we cross paths with people who trigger us, it is all for a reason.

Your triggers are purely lessons for you to learn – because you are here to be a student of yourself and what makes you tick (and also what ticks you off).

> **Accept advice with love and kindness, but don't carry around other people's stuff for them when they throw it at you. You only have to carry your own stuff.**

Mother Teresa didn't
walk around complaining
about her thighs. She
had shit to do.

The Power of Sisterhood

*There is one thing more powerful than
magic, and that is Sisterhood.*

Can you imagine what would happen if women were all as friendly to each other every day as they are when they meet each other drunk in the ladies' room?

**Instead of comparing yourself to other
women, or searching for flaws, be a beacon
of love for all women around you, and
the women you have yet to meet.**

Smile at women in the street. Chat to girls in bars. Why not?

Filled with our own insecurities, us girls often still don't expect genuine love from other girls we have just met. It still seems to take us by surprise when other women want to be friends with us and think we're awesome! So give love out freely to others. In abundance. And knock their socks off with it. Compliment the women you admire. If you think she's beautiful, tell her.

Smile on the train. Compliment her outfit.

Or her hair.

Or just her general beauty!

If you're chatting to a girl and you realize something about her that is a real gift – tell her!

All women need affection. All women need compliments. And let's be honest – a lot of women aren't getting that from their men.

If I see a girl who looks amazing in her outfit, I will go out of my way to let her know. I know she probably spent ages deciding what to wear that day, or what goes with what.

So, if a girl looks fierce, well-dressed, or that colour simply goes *amazingly* with her skin tone – then she should get to hear it said to her. And you might well be the only person to tell her that day. You might just even make her freaking day. And isn't that a beautiful thing?

Spread your love generously among other women and just watch how much love, joy and sisterhood it brings back into your life. Watch how much it makes you appreciate your own beauty, too.

Accept compliments

You're worthy. You know how it usually goes.

> Other girl: 'Oh, I love your dress!'
>
> Us: *'Oh, this old thing?! I've had it years, got it in the sale, it was super cheap.'*
>
> Other girl: 'Did you get your hair done? I love the colour!'
>
> Us: *'Oh yeah I did, but still not happy with it, I might go back and get them to redo it...'*
>
> Other girl: 'Your skin is flawless!'
>
> Us: *'Trust me it's not, I have had loads of spots recently...'*
>
> Other girl: 'You look amazing! Love your outfit!'

Us: 'Thanks, but I feel really fat today, this outfit looked better when I was smaller. In fact none of my clothes fit me right now and I really need to lose some weight...'

Now come on. This is not a way to accept love into your life, Goddess. This is a way to let your fear, doubts, insecurities and Inner Skinny B win. How about trying something that goes a little more like this:

Other girl: 'Oh, I love your dress!'

Us: 'Thank you so much! It's one of my favourites, I got it from blah blah.'

Other girl: 'Did you get your hair done? I love the colour!'

Us: 'I did! Thank you so much for noticing!'

Other girl: 'Your skin is flawless!'

Us: 'Thank you so much, I use this cleanser called blah blah.'

Other girl: 'You look amazing! Love your outfit!'

Us: 'Thank you so much – that means a lot actually because I haven't been feeling my best in it – but that has really made a difference so thank you!'

When you listen to compliments – and truly accept them with love – your life will change phenomenally and you will begin to appreciate your beauty, and the beauty of the Goddesses around you. Even if it feels 'put on' at first, you will always wind up believing the story you are reinforcing to yourself. So keep reinforcing the belief that you deserve those kind words, you are worthy of love, and you are grateful to feel appreciated.

You are more than your body, and so is she

Look deeper than your exterior shell, aka your body, your clothes, your hair, your skin – how about telling your girlfriend what a generous and kind person she is, how smart she is, how much you admire her drive and ambition?

How about telling your mum what a great role model she is or how you really admire how she dealt with a particular situation? How about telling your sister how much you appreciate her good sense of humour and big heart? How about looking into your best friend's eyes and saying to her genuinely, 'Thank you so much for being you. You are one of the most incredible women I have ever met and I am so grateful to have you in my life.'

Express all the love.
Feel all the love.
It is what we are here to do.
Only love is real.

You have a much bigger purpose in this lifetime than worrying about the size of your bum or the backs of your arms. You are here to change the world. You are here to make your mark. You are here to learn how to love.

You can tell who the strong women are – they are the ones building each other up instead of tearing each other down.

Part VI

Feel Your Way to Freedom

You've got to feel
it to heal it.

Focus on the Feels

It's incredibly likely that you have no idea just how *amazing* your body can actually feel when it's nourished, supported and loved.

Imagine if every day, you made choices based on having an incredible-feeling body. Imagine if you put your reflection to one side for a while, and started focusing on making yourself *feel* fantastic, instead of thinking only about how it looks.

How do you want your body to feel?

- Vibrant?
- Alive?
- Energetic?
- Bouncy?
- Free?
- Happy?
- Strong?
- Light?
- Agile?

- Powerful?
- Invincible?
- Ready for anything?
- Awake?
- Focused?

Eat based on how you want to feel

Start focusing now on making food choices to make your body **feel** the way you want her to feel.

There's a big difference between how a food tastes initially – that pleasure sensation on your lips – and how it actually feels in your body an hour later, or how it impacts your mood and the way it makes you feel for the rest of the day, or the next day.

If you're struggling with how you want your body to feel, instead consider the opposite question – how do you **not** enjoy feeling?

Here's my guess for how you **don't** enjoy feeling:

- Sluggish
- Tired
- Lazy
- Lacklustre
- Exhausted

- Stressed
- Heavy
- Bloated
- Stuck
- Lethargic

So now, ask yourself: what foods are you eating that are encouraging these feelings?

> **With each food choice you make a decision on how you want your body to feel.**

So which list are you supporting?

I won't tell you what you *should* eat – as I believe you already *know* what you *should be* eating. Instead I want you to start figuring out *how you want to feel* – and which food choices will support those feelings – and which food choices push you away from those feelings. Make choices every day that bring you another step closer to how you want to feel in your body.

You've heard the saying, 'You are what you eat'. Well, that's totally true. Everything is energy. So what is the energy of the food you're eating?

If you want to feel empowered, happy, vibrant, colourful, then the foods you eat should be supporting this. How? Eat foods that are empowered, happy, vibrant and colourful too!

What you eat has an instant effect on how you feel. It could be that you are not eating any foods right now at *all* that are supporting the way you truly want your future body to feel!

In the same breath, if your future body wants to feel at peace with food, happy, vibrant and free, and right now you're counting calories, restricting yourself, and going hungry, then you are **not** eating for the Future You.

Start eating to support the Future You *right now*. There is no other way to get there. You have to start now. Right this second. Not tomorrow or on Monday. Not next week or next month. Not after Christmas or after your beach holiday. If you have a vision for how you want your body to feel – then you have the power to start eating based on that feeling *right now*.

Fresh fruits, vegetables, green smoothies, fresh juices, nuts, seeds, my homemade granola, coconut, avocado, warm bowls of quinoa, soup, big hearty stews, big abundant fresh salads, herbs and spices, freshly made home-cooked foods. All this food makes my body feel how I want it to feel every single day. So I always try to make choices involving these foods where I can. What about you?

Some of the foods that do not support my vision for how my body wants to feel include dairy – because it makes me feel quite heavy and sluggish – bread, pasta, pastries, refined sugar. Eating meat doesn't sit well with me for ethical reasons, but it also makes my body feel tired – like my body is struggling to digest it and deal with it. Eating processed foods make me feel disconnected from nature. Eating greasy, oily foods makes me feel dirty and unattractive. Eating sugary foods makes me feel empty, like a trash can, and not nourished.

Now – that's not to say that I don't eat these foods sometimes because I do – I believe balance is key – and sometimes I choose momentary pleasure over how my body wants to feel in the long term. I believe we all do sometimes, because we're human.

But if you commit to making small shifts towards your long-term choices and away from quick, short-term tastes, you will gradually do it oh-so-naturally, and you will realize very quickly that your body 'craves' less and less of the stuff that makes you feel yuck. And when you do have those odd times of eating the food that *doesn't* make you feel so good, your body will shout about it and let you know, by way of indigestion, constipation, bloating, diarrhoea, skin breakouts, low energy, stomach aches, etc. And nobody enjoys that. You'll be far more likely to think again next time.

> *It's all down to listening to the*
> *wisdom of your body.*

You truly are what you eat. Tune in to your body and listen to how she reacts to different foods. You can be your own expert, without having intolerance tests, or going to a specialist. **Really, you are the expert of you**. You just need to connect and listen.

Play, experiment, try new foods – you're the boss!

If like most of us, you tend to get stuck eating the same foods over and over again, there could be a whole load of wonderful foods that you're missing out on. And how are you going to know what foods make your body feel great, if you are stuck in the same old patterns?

I'm a big believer in making food fun, exciting and varied. Food is there to be enjoyed – and when it's food that makes your body feel great – what's not to enjoy about that!

So Goddess, be a little more adventurous. Try new foods. See how your body likes them or doesn't. Be your own expert. And observe how your body feels afterwards.

Give yourself permission to have fun with this. Maybe you want to try a new recipe or cook with a new vegetable or experiment with having no meat in your dinner tonight, or seeing how you feel when you don't have a big bowl of pasta, and go for a big fresh salad with avocado, walnuts, beetroot and lentils instead. Maybe you want to take a few foods off your 'fear list', and just see how your body reacts to them instead?

Maybe you want to try having a big fresh smoothie in the morning instead of cooked foods, and see if you notice a difference in your energy levels. Or vice versa! Maybe cooked foods feel much better in your body in the morning than a smoothie does? It's your call.

You may feel more grounded and centred when you have a bowl of porridge in the mornings, **or** it might make you feel sluggish.

You might feel stronger and more grounded when you eat meat **or** you might feel lighter, more energized and happier when you go for a veggie meal instead.

You are the boss, remember. You don't have to play by the rules. You are creating the life you want and you get to choose exactly how your body feels from the foods you eat. You don't have to copy me – just listen to *you*.

Goddess Rachel

'It is impossible to overhaul your life in a week when you've spent so long being a certain way. It's more about taking small steps to happiness.'

At 17 some things happened that I guess sort of defined my life. Before I was OK, pretty happy most of the time and never worried about my weight. Afterwards I was sad, angry, anxious, envious, confused, lost, and desperate to fill the loss with something – and it turned out to be food. Of course, it didn't fill the void and a 4st weight gain left me feeling absolutely miserable.

At 20, I joined a slimming club and lost all of the weight in 122 days. I was ecstatic! I was back to my old self. But deep down I knew I wasn't and the weight loss was just masking what was really going on in my head. Before long I began to put some of the weight back on. Lose it, gain it, lose it. Following one diet or exercise regime after another frustrated me, but the worst part was the feeling of constant failure. I just wanted ONE day where I didn't think about what I was eating while planning my life around 'when I'm slimmer'.

Since finding Mel and The Goddess Revolution, my relationship to food has become much more relaxed. I've always known what is good for me – it's simple isn't it? But not when your body is manipulated by negative thoughts in your mind.

Now I create delicious meals for myself, with things I know are good for me. But at the same time I'm also able to eat things that aren't so good for me and not feel like a failure. Changing my relationship with food, with myself, has also given me a huge self-confidence boost and inspired me to realize my dreams. I've arranged to go travelling and booked to go on a copywriting course – the one thing I've thought about for years but never had the confidence to even enquire about it.

There are still things about my body that I don't like. I still see and poke bits that I really would rather not be there. I still have consecutive days when I don't eat any vegetables. And I think that's OK, because this is a journey and if Mel has taught me anything, it's that it's about growth.

It's Food, Not Religion

OK, so let's talk labels. I'm not talking about ingredients labels here, I'm talking about **diet** labels – by this I mean, calling yourself a vegetarian, a vegan, a pescatarian, Paleo, whatever.

I firmly believe that in order to live a life free from ever dieting again, you need to stop putting these labels on yourself, or feeling like you need to categorize how you eat.

Meals, dishes, recipes can be labelled, sure. *This meal is vegan. This meal is Paleo. This meal is gluten-free.*

But labelling yourself as a person, based on your eating habits, can come with all kinds of pressures and judgements. Judgements from yourself, as well as others.

Because again, you have given yourself a hat to wear – a set of rules to abide by. What happens if one day you decide you want to break a rule? Maybe your body doesn't want those rules for the foreseeable future? If you choose to break one of those rules one day, or even do it by accident, it comes with all kinds of shame, guilt and feelings of not being good enough, or not being able to stick to your label well enough. If you want true food freedom for life, commit to living label-free! You are a unique human being with a unique relationship to food. A unique set of eating habits. A unique body.

I completely respect that a lot of people choose vegetarianism and veganism for reasons that have nothing to do with diet rules. I have a huge amount of respect for this. And I personally feel great from having no meat in my diet and little dairy. Not only does my body feel more energized, but I also feel like I am contributing to a healthier planet, fewer animals being slaughtered and I feel comforted knowing that I am doing what I can to lower my risk of cancer, especially after the death of my father.

However, when I decided to 'go 100 per cent vegan', with my history of dieting behind me – I definitely felt like a prisoner by my own rules. I judged myself constantly if I ever wanted to eat something outside of veganism, like eggs, cheese or fish. I broke my rules and then was mortified about it.

With a diet, with a label, comes guilt and shame.

So, if by labelling yourself you feel like you are placing yourself on a diet, then it's simply not going to work. I'm still always being asked *'what I am'*, but I'm not cool with putting myself in a box like that. So I just say that I don't like to label myself but I eat to make my body feel good – and I personally feel much better not eating meat, eating a lot of plants, and occasionally eating fish. I find that answering this way stops any judgement or debate. After all, nobody can argue with what makes **you feel good**. You're the expert on you, not them.

I personally feel better eating this way, but everyone feels differently. It's a personal choice. Let people eat what they want to eat. We are all eating to do the best we can to nourish our body with the tools we have. It's none of your business how other people do their food, and how other people eat to make their bodies feel good. It's food, not religion.

How to Eat Whatever the F You Want

When I tell people I eat whatever the F I want, they don't believe me. How can this be possible, they ask, picturing me gorging on Oreos and ordering pizza every night?

Well, the answer is simple – *it's knowing what you actually want to eat* in the first place. I want to feel nourished and fabulous. I know which foods make me feel that way. So yeah, I eat what I want!

Trust that your body wants the real food – and the rest comes naturally.

I eat whatever I want. Meaning if I want something, I eat it and I enjoy it. It just so happens that usually what I want is to make my body feel nourished!

I will never again deprive myself of food I want to eat. I know the vision for how I want my relationship with food to be: **Freedom-based**. I drink green smoothies and juices, make delicious veggie chillies and curries, am obsessed with avocados and love a superfood salad.

I also love red wine and a cheese platter, and have a soft spot for bottomless sushi. I am a sucker for lemon meringue pie, and if you take me to a cocktail bar that serves Espresso Martinis, I will be your friend for life.

It's called balance.
Eat what you want to eat, based on the way you want to feel.
But allow yourself to paint outside of the lines.

I am no saint. I don't have a perfect diet nor do I want one. I know I make mainly healthy choices for my body and take ownership over my decisions. And I refuse to punish myself. Most of the recipes on my website are plant-based. All of them are healthy and should encourage you to feel good. You won't find meat in my recipes, nor refined sugar or a lot of dairy. And this is not because I am telling you never to eat these foods but because we simply do not *need* more meat. We do not *need* more sugar or more dairy.

We need more plants, more real foods,
more goodness, more nutrient-dense foods,
more leafy greens and more superfoods.

I don't want you to be perfect. I want you to be OK with being imperfect. I want you to *bask* in your imperfect-ness.

And I want to assure you that I am far from perfect.

I am imperfect just like the rest of the world – there are like seven billion of us imperfect folk wandering this planet. And we all gotta eat.

I love food. And I want you to love food too. People who love food are the best folk, after all.

Goddess Harriet
. . . .

'Now I've freed myself from all the rules, I'm finally seeing my body change – but I still feel more confident now than when I was that perfect size 10 to 12, I just try on clothes and don't worry about the size.'

I had tried every way possible to lose weight – including not eating and bingeing and living off coffee and Red Bull. I'm Type 1 diabetic so dieting has played havoc with my health and I've yo-yo dieted for so long that my wardrobe ranges from a size 10 to an 18. During my nurse training I became so ill through lack of food, I nearly had to give up on my dream.

Two years ago I became severely depressed, experiencing extreme panic attacks and taking a lot of medication. I've had counselling about my eating habits and grief, which is one of my huge triggers, but could never seem to resolve the issue – always wanting that Golden Nugget.

Since finding Mel and the Goddess Revolution, I've got my life back. I can go for a meal, choose what I like, not have the biggest thing then vomit it back up when I'm home or go out and not eat. I have my social life back and look forward to spending time with my family and friends! My confidence is back. I love trying new foods, I do yoga and classes… and I have finally broken up with the scales!

. . . .

Taking Ownership

We have to make so many choices around food, every single day. Imagine how much time and energy we spend thinking about food, dwelling on it, feeling guilty afterwards and regretting the choices we made. Instead of fretting, follow these five simple steps:

1. Take full ownership of every choice you make. Decide what you are going to eat and – whether it is a green smoothie or a slice of cake – *just f*cking own it*.

2. Enjoy every mouthful. Take your time.

3. Then – get over it.

4. Don't carry it around with you all day, thinking and dwelling on it. Don't punish yourself the next day to 'make up for it'. Don't try to reverse it. Don't bitch and moan about it.

5. Just own it. And then get on with your day.

By owning your choices, you will actually be thinking them through more, by default. Try it and see what happens.

Most girls: 'I'll have the superfood salad.'

Me: Turns into a black hole and consumes all matter around me. No one is safe. There are no survivors.

Eating Out Without Freaking Out

Ever feel like it would be, like, *so* much easier to live a healthier lifestyle, if someone didn't invite you out to restaurants or round for a takeaway?

How you deal with eating out is a total game-changer.

I used to either:

1. Go to the meal, and completely abandon the diet I was on. And when I say abandon, wow. I would order three courses and eat 'til I couldn't stand up. And probably just write the rest of the weekend off too because why bother trying to be good again 'til Monday comes, right?

Or

2. Go to the meal, and try *super* hard to stick to my diet. Which would usually result in me ordering an extremely plain salad and being a total misery guts while everyone else tucked into delicious-looking food. I would push the bread basket as far away from me as possible, and avoiding bringing up the

topic of dessert – even though I couldn't stop thinking about how much I wanted that cheesecake on the menu.

If I didn't take either of these options, I would make up an excuse *not to go out*. Yep, I would actually avoid seeing friends in order to stick to my diet. Mighty sad times for me. No fun whatsoever.

Now I have a great relationship with food, I find it *so* much easier to eat out without having a total meltdown or feeling guilty in the slightest. I eat out at least once a week and it's always a gorgeous experience that I really look forward to and enjoy, guilt-free.

Anyone that's ever dieted or tried to 'eat clean' and follow a healthy lifestyle, will know that it can often be difficult to eat out. Even though there are many restaurants providing healthier options on their menus now, it can still feel like a struggle to find a dish that fits in with your requirements and works for you. That's why it's super-important to have a healthy *mind-set* around your dinner dates.

Changing your mind-set

I know eating out can cause a total meltdown for a lot of women who struggle with their food and weight, so I'm going to share with you some of my top tips for eating out without freaking out. There's no formula or set of rules for this. As always, it's about adopting a new mind-set and then letting your intuition guide your choices.

#1 Focus on the entire experience

Rather than just eating the meal, think about it as if you are consuming the whole evening. If you're going out with some friends, then say to yourself, *'You know what? This isn't actually about the food. It's about seeing my friends and catching up. It's* about seeing how this person is doing in her new job. It's about seeing how this person's getting on with her new boyfriend.'

Don't make it all about the food. Make it about the friends, the restaurant, the whole experience. I'm sure in your head, it may *feel* like it's about the food – but the truth is, really it's about spending time with your family or friends, engaging in conversation, being present and catching up.

#2 Feel your way through the menu

If you're already eating a lot of healthy foods, in abundance and without restricting yourself, then what's most likely going to happen when you look at the menu is that you'll be drawn to the foods that are most similar to what you usually eat. Because you know how great those foods make you feel.

So look at the menu and ask yourself, *'How do I want to feel? What dish will bring me closest to that feeling?'* Try a few on for size in your head. *'How will my body feel after eating that food? Will that nourish me, satisfy me, but also leave my body feeling good too?'*

If you've been restricting or controlling your food a lot before the meal then you're much more likely to set foot in the restaurant and be in the mind-set of, *'Sod it – I'm gonna eat a burger, I'm gonna eat a pizza and I'm gonna eat whatever the hell I want tonight because the rules don't apply!'*

So, the key is, on the lead-up to eating out or a special social occasion, just to be balanced! Have lots of great, amazing, fresh foods, then your body will want more of the same when you get to a restaurant. Don't diet or deprive yourself!

What tends to happen for me when I eat out is that I'll be drawn towards meals that are similar to what I'd have at home. I don't bother worrying about which dishes are vegetarian or vegan, or are free from dairy, gluten or sugar, because most restaurant menus aren't so abundant in those things.

> *Instead of looking at what the dishes don't have in them, look at the good stuff that they contain – what they do have. Always focus on the positive.*

Look at which dishes have loads of vegetables, fibre, good fats or protein. You can always order sides, too. Also, don't be afraid to ask the waiter if they can change the dishes slightly. I've often changed something on the menu, just by asking. If you don't ask, you don't get! Usually they can do it and they don't mind! So ask, 'Can I have that without the cheese? Or the sauce? Or can that starter be made into a main dish?'

#3 Listen to your body

If I'm eating out and I know my body wants a salad, then I won't hesitate in ordering the salad. If I eat out and think *'You know what, actually I really want a pizza tonight!'* – then you bet your bottom dollar I'll order a pizza.

Decide on what it is you really want, and then take ownership of your choice. Don't allow yourself to think *'OK, I'll order this pizza and then I'll make up for it by doing two hours in the gym tomorrow or skipping my next meal.'*

Just own that choice! Order it, own it and, when it comes, enjoy every single mouthful. And when you've finished eating it, let it go. It doesn't mean you have to beat yourself up the next day, it doesn't mean you have to restrict the next day; your body will tell you how you feel the next day! It will probably make you feel a bit sluggish and tired, and you will end up being called towards the good stuff again for next time.

#4 A little of what you fancy won't hurt you – ever

If during your normal day, your normal habits, your normal routines you don't eat any bread or cheese, for example, but then you go to a restaurant and you have a little – it's really *not* the end of the world. Obviously if you know you're going to have a bad reaction to gluten or dairy, don't order those things, but otherwise, take ownership, make the choice, stop when you're full, then move on with your life.

#5 Dessert

I used to have such a sweet tooth that I couldn't imagine ever having a meal, and not following it with a dessert. I just *had* to have a dessert. I couldn't leave the restaurant without having one.

I thought that was just the way I was – and would back it up with a BS tale along the lines of, *'That's just me! I love dessert, I have a massive sweet tooth!'* or *'I'm a sugar addict, me!'* but actually, the truth was, the reasons I was so drawn to sugar all the time were both because I wasn't eating a balanced diet, I was always trying to restrict, and I was also turning to sugar when what I really needed deep down was a hug or a cry. As I've got healthier, and included more variety in my diet, and as I've had more good fats and more plant proteins and proper meals that are really nourishing to my body – *and* as I've stopped using food as a comfort tool, I have also noticed the 'sweet tooth' or 'sugar addiction' has evaporated into thin air.

So now if I go to a restaurant, I'm more inclined to have a starter and a main, and then skip dessert. And that's not me being 'good' – that's just a simple case of 'I could take it or leave it – I'm really not that fussed any more!' Which is the most freeing feeling in the world. Abundance. Sometimes I have dessert and share it with someone. Often the idea of a whole dessert to myself is not appealing, because I know how it will make my body feel, and I'm not crazy about that feeling.

#6 Leave the restaurant behind you

By that I mean – *get over it as soon as you leave.* Just because you ate out, doesn't mean you have to slog it out in the gym for two hours the next day or spend tomorrow eating dust.

Your body will tell you how it feels, so the next day if it starts to feel sluggish and tired and a bit rubbish from the food that you ate, that doesn't mean that you have to feel guilty about it.

It just means that you need to listen to your body, and listen to what she wants the next day. Because what she'll be drawn to will be the fresh, healthy, gorgeous, nourishing foods that your body needs to thrive.

Snack Attack

I always get asked questions about what is deemed a 'good' or 'healthy' snack, and am often asked things like,

* 'What's a good snack to take with me on the go?'

* 'What should I eat in between such-and-such?'

* 'What's a healthy snack for me to make and take to work?'

* 'What's a good snack for before the gym?'

* 'How much snacking do you think is right?'

* 'What portion sizes are right for my snacking?'

Now, you should know me well enough by now to know I am not about to give you rules for your snacking. I'm not a fan of rules, in case you didn't get that.

But, I am, however, going to give you some great mind-set tips and shifts around snacking.

When you eat mindfully as I described earlier, you'll notice that you won't actually be called to snack quite so much.

When you apply my techniques for quitting emotionally eating you'll also notice that you won't be called to snack quite so much, either.

Most of the time when we're snacking, it's actually pretty mindless, and we're not really hungry. We're just doing it on the way to work or in between meetings, or just mindlessly grazing while watching the TV or checking our emails.

We get all caught up about what we should be snacking on, but the truth is you probably don't *need* to snack half as much as you think you do.

Portion sizes also matter when it comes to snacking and I often get asked, *'Am I eating too many nuts in the day?'* or *'How much fruit is too much fruit?'*

If you're not paying attention when you're eating – that's how much.

The moment you disconnect from your food, stop listening to your body – and stop paying attention? – **that's** how you should be measuring your 'portion control'. And if you're getting through a jar of almond butter a week, you're probably not eating mindfully. You're probably just doing it on autopilot.

I am not about to insult you. You and I both already know what constitutes a healthy snack. It's a piece of fruit, a smoothie, some avocado, some nuts, some veggie sticks and hummus. It's the food that makes your body feel good, but in a smaller dose with little to no preparation required.

There are lots of healthy recipes for 'treats' on my blog, and they are healthier versions of desserts and sweet treats – made without butter, sugar, margarine or other processed foods. But I think it's really important still to eat these foods as treats, not just everyday snacking. By this I mean raw brownies, energy balls, seed flapjacks, etc.

A really great snack I would always recommend is a simple green smoothie. You can have half in the morning and half in the afternoon if you're experiencing that afternoon slump. A green juice or smoothie is a great thing to drink through the day to stop you needing to spend time worrying about snack attacks.

But, again, just be mindful when you're eating, use my techniques for combatting emotional eating (getting clear on your reasons and how you're really feeling), and you'll notice that you don't *really* need those snacks as much as you thought you did.

The truth is, when you're having nutritious main meals that satisfy you, nourish you, and make your body feel good, you won't be called to snack in between much at all.

We *think* that we need three main meals and two snacks in between, but really we just need to listen more. So if your body doesn't need a snack at 'snack time', don't have one. No rules.

Your Sacred Kitchen

Back when I was cray cray for diets, I was constantly running away from my kitchen. In fact I spent zero time in there whatsoever. I was scared of what might happen if I stood in that kitchen for too long. I was living off processed weight-loss foods such as slimming shakes, protein bars, naked bars and tins of soup.

I wanted to be in the kitchen as *little* as physically possible. I never cooked. I never made anything. My cupboards were always pretty much bare, out of fear. If I had a fully stocked kitchen, I knew I wouldn't be able to control myself and I would binge on everything. Even if I bought 30 raw food bars and told myself I would make them last a week, I would have binged on the lot within 48 hours. So I did my best to keep my kitchen as bare as possible, to stop that from happening.

But did having an empty kitchen stop me from bingeing? Hell no! I just went to shops to buy my binge food. I wasn't doing the inner work, just trying to control the exterior symptoms.

Now, I see how backwards that was.

And now, my kitchen is somewhere I really love spending time. I practically *live* in the kitchen, I feel so happy there cooking up delicious meals and guess what? I don't find myself with my face in the fridge every night looking for answers like I thought I would.

I have worked with many clients who, as I did, have completely detached themselves from their kitchen and live in fear of the fridge.

Maybe they stuck a picture of a celebrity's body up on the fridge door as 'motivation' to stop them going in there, or tried 'hiding' the chocolate biscuits on the top shelf.

Come on, ladies – we know that trick doesn't fool anybody. When you want to react to emotion with food, or binge – and when that feeling takes you over – a packet of biscuits you hid on the top shelf of the cupboard, or a 'skinny photo' stuck to the fridge is not going to stop you.

Your relationship with your kitchen is crucial.

> **Your kitchen is the sacred space in which you create the nourishment for your body to thrive.**

What kind of relationship do you have with your kitchen? What kind of energy are you bringing to this space?

Maybe your kitchen is small, old, full of unused or outdated equipment, or full of clutter. Maybe you share a kitchen with flatmates.

I have had clients that start working with me, and then tell me that they don't like cooking or don't have any time whatsoever to be in the kitchen.

I totally get that time is of the essence and nobody wants to spend their whole life cooking *all the freaking time*. **But,** to cultivate the happiest relationship between food and your body – yes – you are going to have to at least *try* to get into that kitchen. It's not something that you can keep running away from. You need to connect with the food you are fuelling your body with.

So here's how to start making your relationship with your kitchen a priority.

First, start seeing your time in the kitchen, as part of your *self-care*. See it as just as important as washing your face every morning, brushing your teeth and cleaning your juicer out.

**You have to spend the time
to nourish your body.**

You are worth the time it takes.

**We prioritize what matters to us. Is having
a healthy body a priority to you?**

You can't nourish your body by doing the bare minimum in the kitchen. It just doesn't work. Just like you can't take a diet pill and keep eating crap food. There is not a short-cut here. You have to put some effort in.

The good news is, though, it doesn't have to be hard, or stressful, or annoying. It can actually be amazing. It can bring the *joy* back into food.

If food has felt like a stressful thing to you, a chore, or the enemy – then this step is absolutely *key* for you.

Transform your space

Start by decluttering. By making physical space, you will also be energetically making space for new light and love to enter your life, and for a sparkly new relationship with your kitchen to come into your life.

Go through all your cupboards and drawers, clean out your fridge, go to the back of all those cupboards and chuck out all the crappy food that you *know* will not serve your future self. Get rid. Also chuck out all those old tins you'll never use, and those big bags of caster sugar you never bake with. Chuck out all the sauces and condiments that went out of date months ago. Chuck out that old jar of pickled onions. And clean all your cupboards. You will likely be facing some resistance with this part, but if you are noticing resistance, it means you need to do it more!

Then. Think about what really makes you feel happy and fills you up. What brings you joy? Now, bring some elements of *that* into your kitchen, too! Is music on your list? Then let's start playing some music in the kitchen, baby! Is nature and being outside on your list? Then let's go buy a new plant or a bunch of flowers.

Maybe you want to stick some family photos up in your kitchen, or positive affirmations? Photos of the people that you love or your pets. Inspirational quotes that you love. (*No dieting quotes allowed!*) Make it feel like a beautiful place. Keep it clean and organized. Collect recipes and try them out!

Do you see what we're doing here? Making it a place you really feel at home in, and a place that you want to spend time in. I really hope you will commit some time to do this, because it can create huge shifts in your relationship with food.

I worked with one lovely lady recently, who when I asked to do this exercise, told me her oven hadn't worked for six months! I was like... 'Well how can we move forwards, if you aren't prepared to get your oven fixed?' Of course, it was a sneaky self-sabotage, disguised cleverly with, '*I haven't had the time.*'

Another thing you may need to declutter, and maybe replace, will be your kitchen appliances. If you're using a blender that has a really crappy blade or is gathering dust, then get rid and upgrade. Treat yourself by investing in a new one. You are worth the effort it takes you to upgrade your kitchen, Goddess. These are all investments in your health.

Now, this is not about being a perfectionist or having a perfect luxury kitchen with all the latest and most expensive equipment. Oh hell no. This is about having a kitchen that you *enjoy* being in. And why are we going to be in the kitchen? To *play, create and nourish*, my love!

Allow yourself to play!

Think about how children eat. They play with their food. They are adventurous. Their parents always want them to try new things. I want you to start playing in the same way. This is how you are going to cultivate a beautiful playful relationship with your kitchen, and a great environment to nourish your body in. Make a mess. Burn the granola a few times before you get it right. Make too much smoothie so your blender erupts and let it spill all over your kitchen floor. Mess is part of the fun! Play is good. Variety and experimenting is good. Stick on some music and get happy in that kitchen of yours!

See the beauty in experimenting. If you have kids, *involve* them in the fun. Same goes for your partner. Anything you can use and anything that you can make that involves *playing* with food, I highly encourage. I think it is wonderful. Foods like pizza where you pick your own toppings (*there's a great healthy pizza recipe on my website*), fajitas, smoothies, all these things include an element of creation and fun!

Picking your own ingredients also adds an element of improvisation! Making it up and giving yourself that freedom to be a bit more creative with food is absolutely beautiful and, again, it is satisfying to your inner child. So yes – play, create, and make a mess! This is how food will transition from being the enemy to being a playful friend you can have fun with again.

Cook with Love

'Cooking is like love; it should be entered into with wild abandon or not at all.'

JULIA CHILD

Here are my top 10 tips for cooking in a love-fuelled kitchen!

1. **Cook with coconut oil:** You can buy coconut oil from supermarkets or health shops. It comes in a jar. This is the healthiest oil to use to cook with and goes great with any foods. If you need liquid oil, just melt the coconut oil in a saucepan first.

2. **Make double or even triple the recipe:** Freeze leftovers or keep them for lunch or dinner the next day.

3. **Set aside time for preparing food:** If you're short on time, a slow cooker could be your new best friend.

4. **Involve everyone:** Get your family, partner, kids involved in cooking by making it an experience and fun, not a chore.

5. **Plan to make FUN things – not just meals:** Treats, fancy things that spark your interest, stuff that doesn't fit into your mealtimes – just for extra fun and trying new things out.

6. **Organize your kitchen:** If it's easy to find utensils and ingredients, it will make the process much easier. Have a place for your spices, a place for your grains, a place for your nuts and seeds, and so on.

7. **Use big glass mason jars to store food:** They look beautiful, keep your food fresh and make the whole experience feel more luxurious.

8. **Taste as you go:** There is no better way to enjoy the experience of your culinary skills, than to taste as you go.

9. **Play music when you're cooking:** This will help you to relax, get into your creative flow and unwind from your day.

10. **Sing and dance while you're cooking:** Yep, you heard! Again, this is going to get you feeling great about your food, infusing your mealtimes with amazing, happy energy, and you'll enjoy eating it so much more afterwards.

What energy do you bring to your mealtimes and cooking?

Rushed? Frantic? Chaotic? Mindless?

Everything is energy.

When you're cooking or preparing food with the energy of *'I don't have time for this'* or *'This is such a chore'* or *'I'm so stressed out'* – then that is the energy that you are putting into your body. So ask yourself:

❖ How is your energy around mealtimes impacting on the people you live with and eat with?

❖ How do you want your energy around mealtimes to be? And how will that impact on your family?

- How do you want *their* energy around mealtimes to be?

- What is the energy of the food you're preparing?

- Does the energy of your food match the energy of how you want to feel in your body?

Goddess Lindsay

'I was so caught up in self-hatred that I tried everything to change. Shakes, diet pills, low cal – you name it. Not any more. I've realized there is only one Lindsay. She is beautiful even with a few wobbly bits.'

My mum and aunts were always on a diet so being on one too – or worrying when I wasn't – just felt normal. Sexually assaulted when I was 14 – food also helped me cope, to self-medicate, but it was never my friend. I just felt uncomfortable in my skin and believed that if I could make my body the right size and shape then everything else would fall into place and I'd be happy.

When I started working as a long-haul flight attendant, I didn't really pay too much attention to how I was nourishing my body and got used to grabbing something high-sugar to give me an energy boost at work. Then, on my days off, I couldn't be bothered to cook for myself so lived off takeaways. I'd go to amazing destinations but then spend my time comparing myself to others, push away friends and social events and worry constantly about my weight.

I'd get into a diet for a few days and feel happy that I'd lost a few pounds only to put it all back on weeks later. The feeling of 'I'm not good enough for this diet so I'm not good enough for anything in life' would send me into an emotional eating binge which in turn made me ten times worse. It was a vicious circle and it lasted two decades.

Since working with Mel, that's all changed. I know what foods make me feel amazing from the inside, and how it affects my outside. I've worked through my emotional triggers and know how to deal with them. I mindfully eat anything that makes me feel beautiful, bright, colourful and gives me energy. I've stopped comparing myself to others and I've stopped beating myself up. Eating nutritious food makes me feel good on the inside while outside my hair shines and my skin glows.

These days I'm always smiling and my confidence grows that bit more each day. I love discovering new ways of making me feel good about myself, new recipes, new ways to find some self-love and inner peace. And looking after myself is easy: if the food doesn't serve me in a loving giving way I don't want to eat it.

. . . .

Be Your Own Expert

Creating your own formula and becoming your own expert is really about deciding which foods you nourish your body with, and which foods you prefer not to. If you don't take full *ownership* of these choices then you will wind up feeling unsure, judged (*because you are judging yourself*) and are way more likely to experience what you have previously labelled 'bad days'.

So you need to decide *what* makes your body feel the way you want it to feel. And what you *don't* eat because it makes your body feel not great.

In doing this you are deciding what works for you and what doesn't. And standing your ground by taking full *ownership* of these choices.

Here are a few things I have discovered about my own body, and continue to discover, as I continue to become my own expert of *my* body.

❖   It works for me to have a green juice or smoothie most days. That always makes me feel great.

❖   It works for me to have a smaller breakfast and then a bigger lunch.

- It works for me not to eat too much fruit or I seem to get gassy – that's just what my body tells me.

- More than one coffee a day and I get jittery, anxious and bloated.

- I also discovered recently that it works for me to limit rich raw desserts.

- It works for me to have no meat in my diet, but it works for me to have fish.

- It definitely works for me to drink a lot of water.

- It works for me to include goat's cheese and halloumi in my diet rather than eliminate dairy altogether.

- It works for me to eat avocado every single day. I'm also obsessed with it, so…

- It works for me not to snack that much, but have nourishing meals instead.

- It works for me to enjoy a glass of red wine with dinner out sometimes, but if I have it on weeknights at home? That doesn't work for me.

This is what I have found works for me over the last few years, but it is constantly developing, because I am a lifelong student of myself and my body. This is how I support my vision for how I want to feel.

Any greasy food – fry-ups, etc. – definitely does *not* work for my body and is a complete non-negotiable now for me. When I eat greasy food, I feel so lethargic that it is simply *not* worth it to me. Pic 'n' mix is also a non-negotiable for me because I used to be addicted to the stuff, and now I don't even identify it as food, just chemicals.

Please don't copy my list or think I am giving you any type of rules whatsoever. Again – this is what I've found does and doesn't work for *me*. I've compiled these by listening to my body and observing how I feel after eating various different foods. Try it for yourself. You are the student of your body.

Now here's another very important factor. Putting foods on your 'Doesn't Work For Me' list – does not mean you will never ever eat these foods again in your life. Absolutely not. We are just establishing your lifestyle and new, healthy eating habits for your body.

Your daily habits around food should consist of what foods work and make your body feel good.

Crowding Out vs. Cutting Out

Cutting Out is what diets tell you to do – aka cut out sugar, gluten, dairy, meat, etc. Crowding out is what I want you to do instead.

All the food that you've discovered **doesn't** really work for you? Crowd it out by focusing on eating all the foods that you've discovered **do** work for you!

As soon as you say you're going to **cut** out A, B or C then you want it, you can't stop thinking about it, you feel restricted and have made it a forbidden food.

Crowding out works so much better and a lot of my clients have said that when they focus on crowding out rather than cutting out, they have felt like they are eating so much more than they used to! And they can't believe they are actually losing weight, gaining energy and feeling so fantastic at the same time. So yes – this stuff works.

Don't decide you're cutting out sugar or meat forever. Even though I think I probably won't be a meat-eater again, I don't like to say never – because who knows?!

Realize that *you* are in control of what you choose to put in your body. And what works for you now isn't necessarily for ever either.

Goddess Lisa

'For far too long I was searching for happiness in 'things' and food. I now know that I not only need to feed my body but also my mind and soul, which I'd neglected for far too long.'

I've always treated food as a reward and a comfort. If I were celebrating or feeling down or even just bored – I ate. I love food but when my sister was diagnosed with cancer, it scared me into facing my health and diet. I tried all the latest fad diets. The problem was I couldn't resist the lure of unhealthy food. Then I would beat myself up about my bad choices and cheer myself up with more 'treats'. I was caught in a vicious spiral, which affected my mood and made me doubt my self-worth.

Since I found Mel, I've learned respect for my body and the amazing things it has done for me – including bringing my three beautiful daughters into the world! I now give myself the attention I not only need but deserve and that doesn't mean I am selfish or neglecting my family. It means I am a happier person with more energy and I no longer make my wellbeing the last priority.

I'm by no means a saint now nor do I always make the best choices, but I am a work in progress and I am fine with that. I love the concept of crowding out the bad foods with better choices, and both my family and myself are benefiting from that. I have eaten things I never even knew existed before such as kale and quinoa and I have discovered that fresh, healthy food can taste delicious.

Imagine if we obsessed
over the parts of
ourselves we loved?

Part VII

Viva
La
Goddess

Eat like you love yourself.

Move like you love yourself.

Speak like you love yourself.

Act like you love yourself.

Tara Stiles

You Should Go and Love Yourself

We spend a lot of time thinking about relationships don't we?

We obsess about that guy/gal we're dating, completely over-analyse their messages to the point of confusion, worry about our relationships with our parents and siblings, and get annoyed when our friends don't call us back.

We all have relationships that are amazing, and some, not so much.

Which relationship in your life is the warmest, the most nurturing, the most amazing?

Which relationship makes you feel safe, accepted and loved?

Do you have a person in mind?

Is it you?

Our relationship with ourselves is the most important relationship we'll ever be in. You will, literally, be in it for a lifetime, after all!

You've probably stumbled across that idea before whenever it was a pretty quote image on Instagram or a line in *Sex and the*

City – but it's worth more time than a quick *'Ooh, that's so true!'* acknowledgement before moving on...

If I asked you to define your ideal romantic partner, perhaps you'd include words such as trustworthy, loyal, kind, generous, takes care of me, forgiving, understanding...

How many of those traits would you apply to your relationship with *yourself*, exactly as it is right now?

Are you kind and generous with yourself?

Are you forgiving and understanding when you make a mistake?

Every relationship in our lives is a reflection of our relationship with ourselves. Start treating yourself the way you want to be treated, and watch the world move around you. It's actually quite amazing!

Recognize that you are already in the most important relationship of your life right now – the one with YOU.

Work on your relationship with yourself and everything else will make an effortless upgrade.

The greatest love is reserved
for those who dare to
believe they are lovable.

How to Really Love Your Body

'If you want the Goddess, worship her.'
DANIELLE LAPORTE

What does 'self-love' really mean, anyway? Isn't it just some made-up thing people talk about online?

Self-love is the most neglected part of weight loss and health.

I know that without making a commitment to learn to love myself and my body, I would *never* have healed my destructive eating patterns. It would have been physically impossible. I would still be in a daily, ongoing battle with food. I would still be hopping on the scales every morning to determine my mood for the day. I would have remained using my body as a battlefield, not as a home or a friend.

**Learning to practise the art of loving yourself
and your body is absolutely essential if you
want any chance of happiness in your own skin.**

When you hear 'love your body', what do you feel? Do you cringe a little? Roll your eyes? Or think that it couldn't possibly apply to you?

Maybe these questions come up:

* How can I love my body when it doesn't look the way I want it to look?

* How can I love my body and also be trying to change it at the same time?

* How can I love my body when she isn't the weight I want her to be?

* Can't I just like, lose weight first, then start trying to love myself after that?

Self-love is not about abandoning healthy principles and eating just anything instead. Quite the opposite.

Love and respect your body ENOUGH to make choices that make your body feel fantastic.

It's a huge misconception that you'll start loving your body **when** you get to your ideal weight or you're feeling strong and healthy – the opposite is true. You'll get to feel amazing, radiant, strong and vibrant **because** you've been loving your body – and treating it accordingly.

When you love your body, you want to do what's best for her.

You *want* to work out to make her stronger – not to 'get abs'.

You *want* to eat amazing healthy food because of how well and alive it'll make her feel.

Accepting and choosing to love her where she is right now, is all part of the process. Acceptance doesn't mean saying 'F it' and throwing the good habits out of the window.

Your Body Is Your Best Friend

'Loving your body' isn't about looking in the mirror and trying really, really, really hard to love those parts of your body that you've spent years trying to get rid of. Nor trying to make it look like someone else's body – a celebrity's, a girl on Instagram's, or your former 20-year-old self's.

This is the stuff that really sticks.

Treat your body like she's your best friend.
Respect her, honour her, listen to her.

Start to think of her like she's one of your besties. A girlfriend that you have so much love for that you would never disrespect her. You would never want anyone to hurt her, and looking after her and making sure she's safe are of upmost importance to you. Maybe instead of a girlfriend it's your mum, your sister, or your daughter.

Your feelings for her run so much deeper than just what you see on the outside. (Can you imagine if we loved our best friends, mums, daughters purely because of the way they *looked*?! If they gained a few pounds or felt bloated would we suddenly turn our backs on them and disown them?! Of course not, don't be so ridiculous, I hear you cry.)

This love between girlfriends is a real deep love, respect and honour.

This is how we should love ourselves.

This is the love we should have for our body.

It means sticking with your body through thick and thin, listening to her, trusting her innately, respecting her, loving her through and through, and not ignoring her when she's shouting at you. It means being your body's cheerleader when she's feeling rough, and championing her when she's feeling fab.

Loving your body also means not talking down to her.

Would you talk to your daughter, your mum, your best friend in the same way you talk down to yourself?

Talking to ourselves…they say it's the first sign of madness… yet we all do it. Whether you're muttering to yourself while driving or running a subconscious mental dialogue, it's totally normal!

But the important question is how do you talk to yourself?

That little running commentary in your head isn't always kind, especially when you're in certain 'trigger scenarios' – in the shop changing-room, in a mirror, even in the bathtub or just getting dressed in the morning.

Have you ever found yourself insulting your body, or calling yourself names for being lazy, or useless – or berating yourself for still carrying around those extra 10lbs?

Would you ever say those things to your best friend? Of course not!

All those insults and cutting judgements about ourselves and our bodies wouldn't even cross your mind! If you ever spoke to them the way you speak to yourself, they'd probably be so hurt and offended! So why speak to yourself that way?

The longer we talk down to ourselves, the longer we stay imprisoned in body jail, so use the following three steps to upgrade your self-talk.

1. Catch yourself in the act when you are talking down to yourself.

2. Change the script in your head.

3. Be kind, forgive yourself and drown out negative or hateful thoughts with love and compassion. You deserve it and you are enough. Just as you are.

> **You and your body should be working as a team, rather than you fighting against her.**

Goddess Amanda

'It's still amazing to me how quickly I've managed to reverse a lifetime of negative mind-set.'

I'm now 33 but looking back it feels like I spent my twenties consumed by diet rules, exercise DVDs and gym memberships, comparing myself to others and trying to reach my goal weight. Each time, I'd get excited by a new diet, believe it would make me happy, do really well for week or two and then slip, start again... give up! Hate myself, hate the diet... find a new diet and be optimistic and excited again... pattern repeat.

I was always able to put on a confident 'face' to the world and pretend I was happy. But the ugly truth is I didn't like myself. I thought I was fat, ugly and unworthy of friendship or love. A fraud, and one the world would be better off without.

Looking back I know that my self-confidence was non-existent and the self-hatred had turned into something much deeper – depression – but at the time I certainly wouldn't have accepted that fact! I was also pregnant and, when I finally realized, it was like my life imploded. I thought how could I possibly be a mother when I was no use to anyone, so I terminated the pregnancy and told my husband I didn't love him any more and it was over.

That was in May 2014. Fast forward six months and I was back living with my mum, reading lots of self-help books, walking the dog on the beach every day, eating healthily and had started yoga. I understood that the depression had caught me unawares and was open to changing my life. Then, along came Mel, just when I needed her most and I was ready to listen to her message.

Now I don't need to diet or weigh myself at all. I don't analyse myself in the mirror and think mean, horrible thoughts about myself. I don't count calories, and I don't deny myself food groups! I eat lots of fresh, colourful and really tasty food! I've learned new skills in growing and cooking food, and I'm inspired and excited when I open my fridge and cupboards! Listening to my body, I've learned what foods make me feel bad or don't agree with me and I don't go for them.

My husband and I have made amends, too, and are trying again. Couples' therapy really helped us, but I believe the biggest change was my mind-set – my relationship with myself and with food. I learned to love myself, to listen to my body and what she needs and to give it to her!

In doing that, I also found my self-confidence and self-worth, and I am the happiest I've been in all my life! I also now have the happiest marriage because I'm real. I'm true to myself, so I ask for what I need instead of putting someone else's needs first, I have the energy and zest for life back that I'd lost.

My husband and I are trying for a baby now, but my attitude and perspective is so different and I'm ready to embrace any body changes with love.

. . . .

Loving your body is
really about listening and
connecting on a daily basis.

Get a Body You Love by Loving Your Body

When you respect your body, she will reward you with a life beyond your wildest dreams.

For many of us this means undoing a whole lifetime of body obsession or feeling like we are always judged on our appearance. Learning to love your body is something that takes time and daily effort.

***Love your body even if you're not
in the best shape of your life.***

If you're not in the best shape of your life right now, maybe you're struggling to love your body, because you're constantly comparing yourself to how you *used to look*. As a former model I can totally relate to that. I have spoken to athletes and personal trainers who have said the same thing. But it applies to all of us. If you've spent a time in what you consider to be great shape, and now you're not 'there' – it can be a real struggle to convince yourself that you don't need to get back 'there'.

When I was in 'the best shape' of my life – or what I considered to be – I was miserable with how I looked and constantly scrutinizing myself – way more than I do now.

It's completely fine for you to love your body AND want to make your body the best she can be!

The key is to do it all from a loving place to begin with.

Your body now is your body *now*. There is no going backwards, no rewinding the clock, only moving *forwards*. Living in the past or striving for an old version of yourself will always be a losing battle. How can your body best support you *right now*, and indeed, in your future?

> **Only loving your body when she's in the best shape is like only loving your kids when they are best behaved.**

Be your number one fan:

Be proud of yourself.

High-five yourself when you achieve something awesome. (In your mind that is; you don't want to look crazy.)

Tell yourself how proud of YOU you are.

Champion yourself.

Give yourself pep talks.

Be your own cheerleader.

You are one sassy lady.

And you've got this.

Forgiveness

'Without forgiveness, life is governed by an endless cycle of resentment and retaliation.'

ROBERTO ASSAGIOLI

A huge part of loving yourself is learning to forgive yourself, on a regular basis. Particularly if you find it hard to forgive yourself around food choices or hold on to your past choices, and use them as a stick to beat yourself with.

Forgiveness is everything.

Forgiveness is what stops you from feeling trapped by past decisions and experiences, and what truly sets you free.

Forgive yourself for not being perfect, or having it all together. Release the grudge you are holding with yourself, and let yourself live.

Forgive yourself for holding on to past choices around food.

Forgive yourself for shaming yourself, or carrying around guilt or resentment.

Forgive the people around you for influencing your choices, or not being amazing role models to you growing up.

Forgiveness will set you free and begin your journey of self-love.

Be the L'Oreal Girl

'Cause you're worth it!

Do you put off simple self-care rituals, such as having a quiet relaxing bath, getting a manicure or just going to the hairdresser?

Do you avoid asking for what you really want for your birthday and Christmas because '*it's all about the kids anyway*' and it would be *selfish* to think about yourself?

It is *never ever* selfish to take care of YOU.

Nourish yourself, in every possible way, because you can't give to your family, your work or your friends when you're feeling frazzled and depleted.

Not making yourself a priority always has an effect on your health. Once you fall into the bad habit of not making yourself a priority, your eating habits can decline, you stop working out and looking after yourself and even start drinking less water and more coffee. Crazy, right?

**Life hack: You are absolutely
allowed to spoil yourself.**

Realize that you are *worth* the effort. Do things on a regular basis that make YOU feel fabulous, like a Goddess. Buy yourself flowers, wear the clothes you love. Chuck out the stuff that makes you feel crap. You are worthy.

Know this: How you treat yourself is how you are inviting others to treat you.

Other people in your life will notice how you treat *yourself* and then subconsciously respond to it by treating you in the same way.

If you're feeling like you're being taken for granted, ask how you are taking *yourself* for granted. If you're feeling unsupported, ask how you are not supporting *yourself*? It always comes back to your relationship with yourself.

I had a client recently who realized she was making a big effort to be healthy and have good food in the house when her boyfriend was there, or when she was cooking for more than one person – but as soon as it was just her? All that effort went out the window. Now – what kind of a message is that giving your body? It's a message that says, *'You're not worth it'* on your own.

When you start **making** yourself worth it, it has a huge impact on every other aspect of your life. When you cultivate a beautiful relationship with yourself, you become a magnet for other beautiful relationships around you.

But first you have to believe that you are worth it.

Your self-worth is really so important. It is one of the most crucial parts of this book – and one of the biggest things you have to learn in your life in order to grow and heal your relationship with food and your body.

When I was at my worst with my food, guess where my self-worth was? It was on the floor. And because I had zero self-worth, because I was always beating myself up, I also attracted *shitty* boyfriends into my life who lied to me, I attracted *shitty* friends who didn't care that much about me, but this was nobody else's responsibility but mine. It was a mirror for how I felt about myself. Which was? *Shitty.*

And it goes the other way of course – when you respect and value yourself, respect and value your food and respect and value your body, other people will respect and value you too. It's the law of attraction.

You are creating the world you see.

How do you want to be
treated, valued, loved and
respected in the world?

Start with how you
treat, value, love and
respect yourself.

The Divine Responsibility of Self-care

Self-care is my absolute favourite thing, and it's a huge part of you healing your relationship with your food, your body and your self.

Self-care is the art of the Goddess.

Self-care is simply about taking good care of you. Doing things to make you feel wonderful. That might be taking yourself on a little date to a new breakfast place. It might be spring-cleaning your home and making it feel beautiful. It might be lighting candles, running yourself a bubble bath or giving yourself a face mask. Time spent in your kitchen also counts, as does going for a long walk or meditating.

When was the last time you took a day by yourself, to do things that make *you* feel great, by yourself?

Write out some goals and dreams, do some journaling, go get a cut and blow dry just for the sake of feeling fabulous.

The more time we dedicate to slowing down and allowing time for self-care, the less we feel the need to 'fill the space' by grabbing food or mindless eating. And the more time we allow for self-care, the more our relationship with our body grows strong, the more we learn to respect our own boundaries, and can make conscious decisions on where we are deciding to invest our precious time and energy.

This might be a totally scary concept, but it's time for you to prioritize YOU, Goddess.

Your self-care is the time you spend on you, when you're not running around after other people or working your buns off. All those things you think you *would* or *should* do, but never seem to find the time, so never get round to doing. This so crucial to your relationship with food and your body because it forces you to slow down and do things with no specific *goal or outcome attached*, but just because it feels good for you to do.

It's about learning to be comfortable in your own company, which can be hard for some of us. I know it used to be hard for me. Self-care is so much more about '*being*' than '*doing*'.

This used to be such a difficult concept for me but now self-care is something I always make time for. If I have let my self-care slack during the week, I prioritize it on the weekends above anything else. This is again, all about listening to what you really want and need.

The more you do it, the more it will become second nature, and this is going to have a big impact on how and what you eat. When you make more time for self-care, you won't be called to overeat or binge, because your energy will be much calmer and happier. Your food choices should gradually become more purposeful, and more thought through, because you're allowing yourself the time to slow down and be with your body.

Trust me. This works.

It's like a muscle you have to keep working, but once you're in the habit of making yourself worth it, just watch as your life begins to change and click into alignment.

Goddess Kirsty

'I used to be so ashamed of myself... now I take care of myself and it fills me up with joy, and I'm smiling again – dropping four dress sizes is just part of that joy!'

I found Mel after what seems like a lifetime of dieting. By that time I was living on Easter eggs and takeaways, and couldn't walk up the stairs without getting breathless! It wasn't just the extra weight but I didn't take any pride in my appearance and went weeks, months, without eating vegetables. I felt like I was just waiting to get seriously sick.

I made excuses not to go out – even to go shopping – just because I didn't think I'd be able to walk there. I would stand in my kitchen pushing any food I could find into my mouth and crying because I was shoving food into my mouth! Even though I have an amazing husband and two wonderful children I felt sad, lonely and miserable.

Now I'm the healthiest and happiest I've been in a long time. I spend much more time on myself, taking long baths, having my hair done, using quality products on my face and body. I realize the emotion I'm feeling and know how to deal with it in a way that isn't food. I'm no longer sad, lonely, miserable or ashamed of myself. I'm proud of how I've managed to turn my life around!

I still love food but the food I love has changed completely, now that I know what makes me feel good and what doesn't. I don't just eat for the sake of it any more, I eat because I'm hungry and

I haven't had a binge or stood crying in the kitchen at all since meeting Mel in April last year!

I love and respect my body now, I no longer look in the mirror and hate what I see, I love her because she's mine and she's done some amazing things for me, she proudly braves the scars of bringing our two beautiful children safely into the world! My confidence has definitely improved too – I used to put on a front before, so it may not be obvious to others but my confidence is real now – I'm the real ME!

. . . .

Need some self-care ideas? Head on over to www.melwells.com/bookbonuses to download your free Goddess starter kit!

Embrace Your Gifts from Your Ancestors

You become BEAUTIFUL the moment you start being yourself. The moment you start embracing who you are – ALL of you. When you look in the mirror and realize the beauty of every part of you.

Those stretch marks? Tiger stripes. And for every woman who wishes she didn't have stretch marks there is a woman who wishes she had them.

Also, find me a woman over the age of 23 who doesn't have cellulite on her body. Dimples are still beautiful, whether they're on your face or on the backs of your thighs.

Your body is your home – not your battlefield.

Rather than looking in the mirror and choosing to feel disgusted with what you see, choose to be proud of a healthy, strong body that has supported you through thick and thin. Through all the trials and tribulations of your life up to this point.

True beauty is not about how tiny your waist is, how your bum looks in jeans, or about how perfect your skin is. You know this already. Because you know, the most beautiful women you've met have been the ones who are happiest in their own skin.

Beauty is about your aura, your energy, your vibe. Beauty is when your face lights up, beauty is when you laugh uncontrollably.

We've all met women who have this absolutely amazing confidence and just are so comfortable in their own bodies, right? They are totally rocking it and they know it and we know it and everyone knows it!

I used to want to change my shape so badly. I thought if I lost enough weight then I was bound to change my body shape and suddenly have a small waist. And I got so skinny, and guess what, nope, my body shape did not change. I just had a smaller frame. It was still *my* frame. My bones didn't shrink.

**You are 50 per cent your mum
and 50 per cent your dad.**

**Your unique body shape is a gift
passed down from your family.**

**Every part of your body is a little
gift from your ancestors.**

Babies are not born with excess weight. They are all the same. What happens is just conditioning, environment, experiences. All of which contribute to your unique relationship with food and your body.

Work out because you
love your body, not
because you hate it.

Work Out Like
a Goddess

Stop looking for abs in the mirror after every workout, and start paying attention to how you *feel* during your workout and after!

Moving your body in the right way for you makes a huge contribution to how you feel living in your body. And yet so many of us avoid exercising, or use exercise in a hateful way, to punish or manipulate our body.

Work out because it feels great to move your body, and keeps her agile, strong and healthy.

Work out because it gives you a rush of endorphins, lifts your mood immediately, helps you sleep better at night, and provides you with massive surges of energy.

Moving your body on a regular basis sends a huge signal to your body that you want to keep her active, playful and strong.

You don't have to go to the gym and slog it out on the treadmill in order to be fit. You also don't have to become a gym bunny over night and have washboard abs to be fit. Just move your body in a way that feels good. Regularly.

Only do exercise that you actually enjoy.

If you're forcing yourself to go to the gym every day, you're always looking for excuses to get out of it, you're not enjoying it and it's making you miserable, then it's simply not going to last. You won't stick to something that you have to force yourself to do.

Try different forms of exercise 'til you find something you LOVE.

Maybe it's swimming, dancing, running, kickboxing, Pilates or CrossFit. Permission to dabble is hereby granted. If you don't know what kind of style of working out you enjoy, try a few different things and see what makes you want to go back for more!

Everything you try will help bring you closer to yourself.

And remember that rest days are just as important as training days. You can't exercise every single day – rest days are totally crucial to all top athletes as well as you! Going hard every day is no good for your body, and doesn't make it feel loved. Love your body by giving her time to recover and rest.

Happiness is the best-kept
beauty secret of all.

Your Goddess Wardrobe

How you decorate your body has a direct effect on how you feel living in it. Just like how you decorate your home. So pay attention to how you dress your body, as well as what you put inside it.

Your body IS your home.
It is the only home you will live
in for the rest of your life.

There will be some stuff in your wardrobe that is energetically keeping you stuck in the past and at war with your body. There are likely some clothes you're going to need to throw out.

Go to your wardrobe and pull out anything that is a good one or two dress sizes away from where you are now. How does holding on to those clothes make you feel?

What memories do you have associated with wearing those clothes? What energy are those clothes holding for you by staying in your wardrobe?

Did you feel vibrant, alive, healthy, all the words you realized you wanted to feel in your own body – when you wore these clothes?

Or were you on a strict diet that made you feel trapped, insecure, consumed?

I had to throw out a lot of old dresses that were beautiful, but a size that I knew, deep down, I wouldn't be going back to anytime soon if I wanted to remain healthy.

So, I got rid. All they were doing in my wardrobe was holding the space and energy of the unhappy thin girl obsessed with dieting that I used to be. I decided I needed to clear it, to make space for the healthy, vibrant woman I wanted to be in the Future Me, and for the rest of my life.

Likewise, let go of any frumpy clothes that make you feel rubbish. Your clothes should make you feel like the best version of YOU that you want to be. They should bring about the energy of how you want to feel about yourself. In the Future You!

Stop buying clothes that are too tight. Stop buying clothes purely because of the label size. Biggest mistake ever. You have to FEEL good in your clothes above anything else.

If you're facing some resistance about chucking out clothes that you **might fit into one day**, then guess what? If your body *is* that size again one day – you will want to go out and buy a whole new wardrobe to celebrate! You won't want to wear the old clothes. And you deserve not to be wearing clothes from years ago! *You are worth it.* Regular clear-outs are worth it. Throw out the old Bridget Jones pants, and treat yourself to new lingerie that makes you feel like a Goddess.

If you can't bear the thought of shop fitting-rooms (designed to make even a Victoria's Secret model have a meltdown), then order online, and when the clothes arrive, try them on with your favourite music playing!

Change the dress to fit your body.

Don't change your body
to fit the dress.

Showing Up and Doing the Work

Treat your self-care appointments with yourself like important business meetings. Do not stand yourself up. Show up for you – every day of the week.

Remember, Goddess – this is a practice that you can live by for the rest of your life. There is no six-week plan here, nor a start and finish date. You will never be 'done' with this. This is a constant practice of observing and connecting with your body.

You are accountable to yourself.

When you support yourself, you will be supported.

You will never find the time to do this work.

You must make time.

Nobody is going to move into your house, cook for you, set reminders in your phone to go and meditate, or force you to connect with your body on a daily basis.

It's up to you, Goddess. You owe it to yourself. And your body is waiting.

From One Goddess to the Next...

If this book resonated with you – please pass on the recommendation to another Goddess in your life.

It is imperative to spread the words of self-love, anti-dieting and positive body image with women worldwide.

After all, there are millions of us still fighting the long, hard fight with food and our body.

You can help spread the revolution far and wide.

If there is a Goddess in your life who needs this message – make it known to her.

You never know, it might change her life.

Goodies!

Want to really immerse yourself in The Goddess Revolution? Oh good!

I've piled together some awesome free goodies for you to go get for free at:

www.melwells.com/bookbonuses

To find me on t'internet:

Pay me a visit at: www.melwells.com
Facebook: facebook.com/iammelwells
Instagram: @Iammelwells
Twitter: @iammelwells

And if you want to take things that step further – to dive deep into your relationship with food, with support from me and hundreds of other Goddesses along the way – join my online Academy at:

www.thegreengoddessacademy.com

I also run luxury Goddess retreats in the UK and around the world, for a total break and real time for you.

Find everything at **www.melwells.com**

Acknowledgements

For my Dad Andrew, who always kept me safe and now continues to do so from a different room. Without you and your constant guidance, this book could not have even been imagined.

For Jackie, Shaun and Charlie who have loved me at my worst, my best, and everywhere in between. Thank you for your unwavering support.

Thank you to Amy, Julie, Sandy, Michelle and the amazing team at Hay House UK, and Reid at Hay House US, for believing that the revolution is here and allowing me to share this message far and wide.

To my fabulous agents Peter and Annette and my incredible Goddess squad, who support this mission every day behind the scenes – Amber, Ros, Ruth, Bry and Joana. You are each invaluable to me.

Most of all, thank you to my Goddesses – far and wide. For my Academy Goddesses, my Retreat Goddesses, my Facebook and Instagram Goddesses, and the Goddesses who have been with me since the very, very beginning.

Thank you to every Goddess who has been called to pick up this book. You make my heart so full.

ABOUT THE AUTHOR

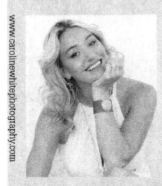

Mel Wells is a coach, speaker and the founder of the blog The Green Goddess Life. Previously a soap actress, Mel struggled with eating disorders for over six years, and created a unique method to heal herself and transform her attitude to food and her body. She now dedicates her time to helping thousands of women worldwide ditch the dieting for good, make peace with food and love their healthy bodies in all the right ways, so they too can reclaim their lives. Mel coaches women one-on-one and also through her online Academy and luxury Goddess Retreats around the world.

 iammelwells

 @iammelwells

 @iammelwells

www.melwells.com

HAY HOUSE
Look within

Join the conversation about latest products,
events, exclusive offers and more.

f Hay House UK

🐦 @HayHouseUK

📷 @hayhouseuk

🖤 healyourlife.com

We'd love to hear from you!